Patient Teaching
and
Communicating
in an
Information Age

HEALTH PROGRAMS

Patient Teaching and Communicating in an Information Age

Carolyn Anderson, R.N., B.S.N., M.A.
Assistant Professor Emeritus,
University of Arkansas at Little Rock,
Department of Nursing

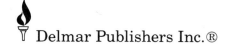

Delmar Publishers Inc.®

NOTICE TO THE READER

Dedication

To: My husband, Jack, for his patience, and my children, Michael and Jackie, for their encouragement and support.

Delmar Staff

Associate Editor: Leslie Boyer
Project Editor: Carol Micheli
Managing Editor: Gerry East
Production Coordinator: Larry Main
Design Coordinator: Susan Mathews

For information, address Delmar Publishers Inc.
Two Computer Drive West, Box 15-015
Albany, New York, 12212

Printed in the United States of America
Published simultaneously in Canada
by Nelson Canada,
A Division of the Thomson Corporation

10 9 8 7 6 5 4 3 2 1

Library of Congress Cataloging-in-Publication Data

Anderson, Carolyn, 1923–
    Patient teaching and communicating in an information age / Carolyn Anderson.
        p. cm.
    Includes bibliographies.
    ISBN-0-8273-3433-8 (pbk.)

    1. Patient education. 2. Nurse and patient. I. Title.
    [DNLM: 1. Communication—nurses' instructions. 2. Nurse-Patient
Relations. 3. Patient Education—methods—nurses' instruction. WY
87 A545p]
RT90.A53 1990
610.73'06'99—dc19
DNLM/DLC
for Library of Congress   89-1317
                                                                                            CIP

Contents

Preface

This text emphasizes the role of the nurse as communicator. This is not an in-depth study of communication but a look at communication as applied in nursing. The role of the nurse as patient teacher is included, since teaching is an integral part of nurse-patient communication. The practical application of principles of communication and teaching is the primary focus throughout this text.

Unit I centers on nurse-patient communication. The process of communication, including verbal and nonverbal aspects, is presented. One chapter deals with human relations development with special emphasis on the importance of listening in building helping relationships. Specific techniques to facilitate communication are discussed with suggestions for application in class activities. Discussion of blocks to effective communication helps the student to be aware of and avoid these responses. Application of communication techniques includes interviews and the recording of verbatim communication interactions with patients. Assessment of the patient and goal setting is integrated in discussion of nurse-patient interactions. Whereas the majority of examples and exercises deals with the average adult patient, one section includes the application of communication techniques in interactions with children and patients who are elderly, are sensory impaired, or have other special needs.

The second unit looks at the role of the nurse as patient teacher. The application of the basic principles of teaching/learning to the individual is the primary focus of the unit. Assessment of the patient is emphasized in determining the best approach to teaching. Adaptation of teaching strategies to the content and the use of teaching adjuncts or aids is covered. A form is suggested for recording the assessment, planning, implementation, and evaluation of patient teaching.

The last unit concerns communication with health care personnel, which is essential in providing adequate health care. It deals briefly with communication within the health care facility, the organizational chain of command, and communication etiquette. There is a short discussion of the dynamics of group interactions. This unit includes documentation of patient care as an aspect of communicating with health team members. The principles of charting are stressed, and methods of recording nurses' notes are discussed, but no one charting method is advocated. Numerous examples of charting and situations for charting are included.

The purpose of this text has been to present readable material in the areas of communication considered to be essential in basic nursing: nurse-patient interactions, patient teaching, communication with health team members, and documentation of patient care. This book is designed to give the student an understanding of basic principles of different facets of communication that can be readily applied in the clinical situation. An attempt has been made to keep the material general enough to be adaptable to any health care facility.

Learning objectives and a glossary of terms with applicable definitions are noted at the beginning of each chapter. Activities to reinforce the content are within each chapter for students to "check on it." There are chapter summaries, brief review questions, and further activities at the end of each chapter to encourage active student participation in the learning process.

ACKNOWLEDGMENTS

There are many to whom I owe thanks for the development of this text. The reviewers contributed enormously in the preparation of the manuscript. Each comment was carefully considered, and most have been incorporated into the text. I gratefully acknowledge the suggestions of the following reviewers: Carol Rosenlund, Weber State College Nursing Department in Utah; Margaret Darnell, Indiana Vocational-Technical College, Indianapolis; Skip Menikheim, Minnesota State Board of Nursing; and Maxine Parks, Odessa College Department of Nursing, Odessa, Texas.

A very special thanks goes to Leslie Boyer, Executive Editor with Delmar Publishers Inc. for her assistance and encouragement. Also thanks to Carol Micheli, the Production Editor who put the final touches on the publication.

I would also like to express appreciation to Ann Larowe, Charlene Bradham, and Mary Jane Miller, my colleagues at University of Arkansas at Little Rock. They "planted the seed" by pointing out the need for a comprehensive communication text and supported my efforts.

Many thanks to the photographer, W. Robert Kane of Little Rock, who patiently cooperated in capturing the desired effect in each photo. I am indebted to the institutions who allowed us to use their facilities and to the personnel who assisted with the photo sessions: to Kaye Mills at Presbyterian Village in Little Rock who graciously assisted and supported our efforts; to Ann Larowe for allowing photographs to be taken between classes at University of Arkansas at Little Rock; and to Pat Hatcher for her assistance at St. Vincent Infirmary Medical Center in Little Rock. A special note of appreciation is extended to all of the individuals who consented to be photographed.

Nurse-Patient Communication

1

The
Communication
Process

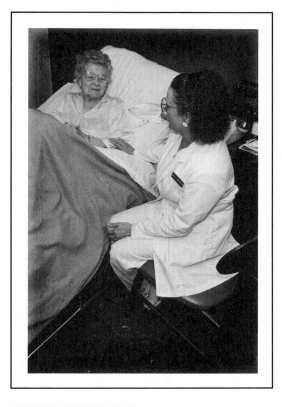

There's a great power in words if you don't hitch too many of them together. **Josh Billings**

OBJECTIVES

Upon completion of this chapter, the student will be able to:

- define the nature of communication.
- describe the normal development of language and communication.
- note influences on language and communication development.
- identify the components of the communication process.
- discuss requisites of effective verbal messages.
- state the effects of paralanguage on the verbal message.
- compare verbal and nonverbal communication.
- list methods of conveying messages nonverbally.
- note the influence of the physical setting on communication.

- list categories of personal space.
- state the effect of frame of reference on communication.
- discuss the importance of feedback.
- note possible interferences in the transmission of a message.
- recognize incongruences in verbal and nonverbal communication.
- explain the importance of therapeutic communication.

GLOSSARY OF TERMS*

Decode   To translate the message into information that is meaningful to the receiver.

Encode   To translate the mental message into symbols that convey the intended meaning to the receiver.

Feedback   The verbal or nonverbal response of the receiver to the message of the sender.

Frame of reference   How a person or event is viewed by an individual based on his or her own past life experiences and current status.

Incongruences   Incompatible items in communication messages that are transmitted simultaneously; verbal and nonverbal messages with different meanings.

Interference   Any external or internal factor hindering the transmission and interpretation of a message as intended by the sender.

Language code   All of the elements in the speech and nonverbal accompaniments used by a person in communication.

Paralanguage   Vocal cues other than words that modify the meaning of the verbal message or communicate meaning without words.

Proxemics   The study of spatial needs of people in their environment and interactions with others.

Stimulus   The idea or event that acts as an incentive to formulate a communication message.

Therapeutic communication   Planned nurse-patient interactions directed toward meeting psychosocial needs of patients.

Transmission   The method by which a message is sent.

*Definitions applicable to content.

INTRODUCTION TO THE COMMUNICATION PROCESS

Communication is the essence of all of our relationships with other people. Through communication people experience happiness and joy; they share ideas, experiences, and knowledge; and they learn what is acceptable or not acceptable in relationships with others. Misunderstandings and broken friendships, as well as many of the everyday problems that occur in both social and workplace settings, can result from lack of communication or from miscommunication. But what is meant by communication?

Definition of the Nature of Communication

A workable definition of communication that is applicable to the nurse as communicator must be established. Webster defines communication as a process by which messages are exchanged between people through a common system of symbols, signs, or behavior. The message may be information, thought, or feeling. The process is successful when the message is transmitted so that it is satisfactorily received and understood. Numerous other definitions are found in the literature, some lengthy and involved, others short, many technical. For clarity and simplicity, Webster's definition will be used.

Communication as a Process To say that communication is a process indicates that it is dynamic. It is ongoing and ever changing, a continuous sequence of events. Contact with others always has an impact on both people involved. This effect may be positive or negative. It is sometimes subtle and sometimes profound and lasting. Communication involves the reaction of each person to the response of the other. Communication continues to evolve, changing with each response, until it is brought to a conclusion.

The Exchange of Messages Between Individuals The two key elements in communication are people and messages. Messages are all of the things people want to share with others. Some messages may be considered more important than others, but each is important in human relationships. The term "message" encompasses all of the interactions between people, from a cheerful "Good morning" to an emergency "Code Blue" call over the intercom for the CPR team. Communication as defined requires satisfactory receipt of a message, so it requires at least two people.

A Common System of Symbols, Signs, or Behavior The process of communication requires that the persons involved have some kind of common language composed of signs or symbols. Without the symbolism of words, communication is extremely difficult. But a common language involves much more than the basic words. Even words have different meanings. The word "frog" may call to mind several things—a small amphibian that jumps, a frog in the throat, a fastener for a garment, a holder for arranging flowers, or a lump on the arm from a sharp blow. Though both persons may speak English, vocabularies and general backgrounds may be so dissimilar that true communication is difficult. The image varies with the background of each as well as the current situation. A person may speak the language of another country but may not be able to communicate if not familiar with the slang expressions. Even within a country, the colloquialism will vary in the different regions.

Messages of Information, Thought, or Feeling The message may consist of information, questions, ideas, dreams, hopes, anger, or frustrations—any of the myriad thoughts that dart through the mind or feelings that are in the consciousness. Messages may be intended to share feelings of warmth, caring, friendship, or love or to convey an attitude of animosity or unfriendliness. The message is whatever is conveyed to the other person by verbal or nonverbal means.

Transmission of The Message Transmission occurs in many forms. It may be direct or indirect; it may be a verbal exchange, a letter, a poem, a song, a gift, a picture, or a message through another person. It may be the actual context of the communication or what is "read between the lines" (whether correctly or incorrectly read). It may be things left unsaid. But transmission remains an important element in the communication process. How the message is transmitted can be an important factor in the effectiveness of communication. Depending on the circumstances, a telephone call, face-to-face communication, or a letter can be the most effective means.

Satisfactory Reception or Understanding of The Message

"I know that you believe
that you understand
what you think I said
But I am not sure you realize
That what you heard is
not what I meant."

The concept of the message being satisfactorily received involves the idea of a common system of symbols, signs, or behavior. However, the understanding of the message involves more than a common system of symbols. It also is dependent on the physical and emotional state of the individual to whom the message is sent. After a bad morning, a cheery "Have a good day" may be answered with a snarl. The message itself was intended to be friendly; however, the individual's emotional state prevented satisfactory receipt of a message of good will.

As noted, communication is a process by which messages are exchanged betw'en people through a common system of symbols, signs, or behavior. The message may be information, thought, or feeling that is transmitted so that it is satisfactorily received or understood. This is a simple definition, but one on which the student can build effective interpersonal communication with patients.

Development of Language and Communication

Since communication is a basic component of human relationships, a brief look at the development of communication abilities and some factors that influence language development will increase the general understanding of communication. In a broad sense, language includes the use of signs, sounds, gestures, or marks having understood meanings to communicate ideas or feelings.

Normal Development of Language and Communication

The development of language is a very complex and involved process. Many studies have been devoted to this topic, and numerous theories have been proposed. The way in which infants progressively develop a method of effectively communicating with others will be dealt with in the following paragraphs.

Infants sometimes announce their arrival in the world with a lusty, undifferentiated cry. This cry soon expands into a repertoire of cries to signify varied wants and wishes. Mothers soon learn to recognize the differences and can usually determine the cause of the vocalization. Within a few weeks the infant finds that sounds other than cries are possible and begins to entertain self and others with varied cooing sounds. By 6 months of age a number of sounds are strung together using different pitches and rhythms in what is termed babbling. The patterns and inflections seem to be an imitation of what is heard.

While still in the babbling stage, the infant begins to develop a receptive vocabulary, a passive understanding of certain words that are frequently used. This passive understanding forms a basis for active speech, which becomes evident when the infant reaches 10 to 12 months of age. Communication starts with use of a single word to indicate an entire sentence or a complex idea. Gradually words are put together. Two-word sentences, which characterize the speech of the 2-year-old child, are primarily in the present tense. Questions are signified by use of inflection. For example, "My doll" may be a question, "Is that my doll?", or a statement, "That is my doll." The intonation used signifies without a doubt what the child means.

By age 4 or 5 years the child has an amazing grasp of grammar. He or she has learned to deal with increasingly sophisticated structures in the language, including compound and complex sentences and phrases within a sentence. The child's semantic development—the increasing understanding of the meaning of words—continues for many years. Language development progresses from concrete to abstract ideas. A child can readily grasp the idea of fairness by taking turns with playmates or the idea of obedience by following the rules, but the terms justice and compliance have little or no meaning. A child is concerned with the here and now, with things that can be seen, heard, touched, or actually experienced. Only with further growth and development can abstract ideas and future consequences of actions have meaning for the child.

Primary Influences on Language and Communication Development

Numerous factors, such as sex of the child, intelligence, whether or not the child is a twin, number of siblings, chronological place among siblings, and bilingual families, influence language development. However, the primary influences are parental stimulation and the socioeconomic and sociocultural status of the family.

Parental stimulation is one of the more important influences on the development of language. Parental interaction includes other adults who are in close contact with the child. Talking to and reading to a child at a very early age provide auditory patterns for imitation, thus stimulating language development. Children whose parents speak a foreign language exclusively may have difficulty with the English language. The Southeast Asian population has recently increased in many parts of the United States. Some of these parents continue to speak their native language and encourage their children to do the same. This is true of Spanish-speaking parents in some areas. While this poses obstacles for some children, others are bilingually fluent.

An important aspect of communicating with young children is the usage of exact terms and correct grammar. While the child's mispronunciation may be humorous, repeating the word incorrectly only reinforces the improper use. This is not suggesting that all incorrect forms of speech should be corrected when a child is learning to talk, only that correct forms should be used when communicating with the child. The parent can encourage the child to be a good listener, because much can be learned by listening at any age. Listening to the child and being noncritical of what is said will accomplish more toward the development of effective listening habits than any amount of lecturing.

Socioeconomic and sociocultural components play an important part in language and communication development. The influences of home, peers, teachers, and other adults are reflected in the language code of the child. Language code refers to the words used, the grammar, the length of sentences, pronunciation, enunciation, the abstractness of terms, colloquialisms, intonations—all of the elements in a person's language. Cultural differences reflected in speech raise the question of whether one style is "right" and another "wrong," the question of standards by which language is evaluated. The term "standard English" may be taken to mean grammatical structures and usages presented in basic textbooks used in the average school system in this country.

The language of the underprivileged may be considered by some to be underdeveloped and substandard. Others will assert that English has a variety of dialects, each being acceptable. Over 20 years ago, Basil Bernstein (1966) proposed a set of distinctions between the language of economically lower-class and middle-class persons. The language of the lower class was called "restricted" because it is shorter and simpler and deals more with concrete than abstract terms. The language of the middle class was termed "elaborated" because the same thought would be expressed in lengthier sentences with more abstract terms and more cause-and-effect statements. The terms "standard" to indicate the elaborated code of the middle class and "nonstandard" to denote the restricted code of the lower class are frequently considered acceptable. These nonstandard English variations have been found to be structured, consistent systems and not forms of English with random errors.

While nonstandard English forms cannot be considered deficient, the child using these forms can be at a disadvantage in the classroom where standard English is the norm. This also holds true for the adult in the workaday world. New usage should be taught without condemning the old. The transition to what is termed standard becomes increasingly important as a technological society places more emphasis on specificity of terms and ability to communicate precisely.

Components of the Communication Process

The communication process in the health care setting takes place within a framework similar to that of the nursing process. The nursing process is a scientific approach to patient care. The first step is assessment of the patient, followed by analysis of the data to serve as a basis for a plan of care. The plan is put into action and the nursing interventions evaluated. The evaluation may lead to reassessment and alteration in the plan. Thus it is an ongoing process. Communication, likewise, is active and ongoing. Although the communication interaction is not always planned in the same detail or in writing as the nursing process is, assessment is essential to determine the best approach to effective communication. The nurse must consider patient responses and make any indicated changes in approach in order to meet current patient needs and promote the communication process.

Communication is an active, ongoing process that can best be represented as a circle. When drawing a circle, there must be a beginning when a mark is first made. This is analogous to the person initiating the communication. The line made can be retraced without lifting or changing direction of the marker. When looking at a circle, who can say where it begins and where it ends? Communication must have a beginning and an end, but during the process, there are no stopping points.

The person who originates the communication is designated the sender. At this point the other person is the receiver of the message, but the roles are constantly being reversed as the communication proceeds. The participants in Figure 1-1 are labeled "A" and "B" to emphasize the fact that both fill dual roles as sender and receiver. This concept is essential if communication is to be viewed as a process.

Although people and messages are the essential in the communication process, other components, such as stimulus, encoding, transmission, and decoding, must be identified to gain a better understanding of the process. These components are illustrated in Figure 1-2.

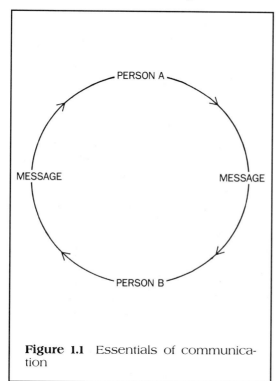

Figure 1.1 Essentials of communication

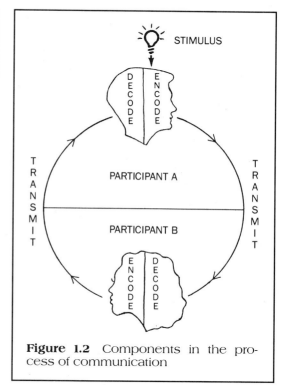

Figure 1.2 Components in the process of communication

Stimulus

A person has an idea, which is the stimulus to initiate communication. This may be a fact to relate to another person, a feeling to share, a question to ask, a concept to explore, or a favor to ask. This idea must be put in a form that can be communicated to the other person.

Encoding

Encoding is the translation of the mental message into symbols that convey the intended meaning. In other words, encoding is simply putting thoughts into words or some form that another person can understand. These symbols represent persons, things, feelings, or concepts. They are usually words, but they may be unspoken.

These symbols do not have universal meanings, a problem that often causes communication difficulties. To encode messages effectively, the following must be kept in mind:

1. A word can mean different things to different individuals.
2. Nonverbal behaviors can alter the verbal message.
3. The message may be expressed in more than one way for clarification.
4. The background and language ability of the receiver must be considered when encoding a message.

The sender must know something of the receiver to encode a message that will be correctly understood. Communication breakdowns can result at this point in the process if the message is conveyed by symbols that are interpreted in a different manner by the receiver than the sender intended.

Transmission

Transmission simply means sending the message. After mentally encoding the message, the sender must consider the method of transmission, the vehicle to carry the message. Transmission may be in any form that can be experienced and understood by one or more of the receiver's senses. It may be accomplished by verbal or nonverbal methods or a combination of the two. Verbal messages may be influenced by factors such as tone of voice or facial expression as well as by the accompanying nonverbal communication. A touch on the arm or holding a hand may convey more of a caring attitude for the patient than expressing concern by words alone. A genuine smile can convey more than many words.

Verbal transmission is not limited to spoken words. The message may be in the form of a letter, a greeting card thoughtfully chosen, a poem written for another, or a song request on the radio dedicated to someone. Regardless of the form of transmission, once the message is sent, it cannot be retrieved. If a message is sent in writing, there is nothing but the words on the page for the receiver to interpret. In face-to-face communication, unspoken "symbols" are part of the encoded message.

Decoding

Decoding is the translation of the message into information meaningful to the receiver—the interpretation of the message. The message may not be decoded as the sender intended for various reasons, such as different connotations of the actual words, nonverbal behavior, or divergent backgrounds of participants. Factors outside the message itself may influence the decoding. The sender may remind the receiver of a person in the past, a memory that will color interpretation of the message. The effect may be positive if the receiver is reminded of a favorite friend or negative if reminded of a person who is disliked. The current physical or emotional state of the receiver will have an effect on what meaning is given to the message. If a person is not feeling well or is emotionally upset, any hint of criticism, though not intended as such, may provoke tears or anger.

Stimulus, encoding, transmission, and decoding complete half of the circle of communication. The message serves as a stimulus for the receiver, and the roles of sender and receiver are then reversed. The circle is completed.

FACE-TO-FACE COMMUNICATION

What tends to come to mind when the term "face-to-face communication" is used is what people are saying to each other. But there is much more to the process than mere verbal exchanges. The way something is said is just as important as what is actually said; a rapid-fire delivery communicates urgency, while a slower delivery may provide reassurance. The optional vocal effects (such as tone of voice) that accompany or modify words also communicate meaning. Nonverbal communication as well as the setting or situation in which the interchange takes place must be considered.

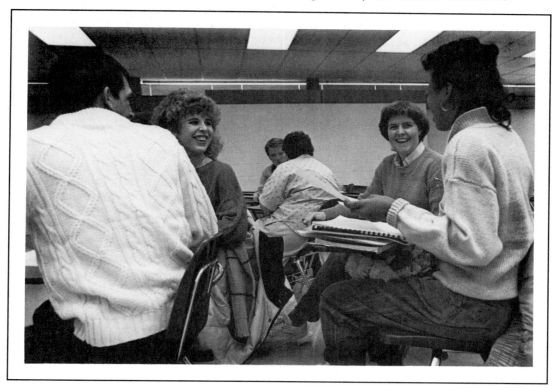

Requisites of Effective Verbal Messages

Effective verbal messages have the following qualities: simplicity, brevity, clarity, appropriate timing, relevance, adaptability, and credibility.

Simplicity. The simpler the message, the less room for misinterpretation. Consider the following:

> *Patient:* What did the doctor mean by a GI series?
> *Nurse:* It is a radiologic study to determine if there are any abnormalities in your gastrointestinal tract.

A simpler and more understandable explanation might have been:

Nurse: It is an X-ray examination of your stomach and intestines.

The concept of simple verbal messages is especially important in dealing with hospitalized patients. Illness lowers the energy level, making it difficult for the patient to comprehend complicated messages. The message should contain all of the necessary information in simple terms.

Brevity. The message should be brief and to the point. Rambling explanations can be very upsetting to patients needing information. For example, Mr. Bloom is scheduled for an X-ray examination in the morning and wants to know when the examination will be completed so that he can visit with his wife.

> *Mr. B.:* When will those X-rays be completed tomorrow?
> *Nurse:* Well, let's see. The technicians start work at 7 o'clock, but you won't go down that early because they have to get their equipment ready. Since you can't have breakfast until the examination is completed, you'll be one of the early ones. It will take about an hour.

Hopefully, this is not a typical reply by a nurse.

Clarity. Messages must contain as many details as necessary to clarify what is meant. Nurses may confuse patients by using medical terms with which patients may not be familiar. To avoid confusion, all necessary details and explanations must be included to make the communication clear and free from misinterpretation.

The number of initials and abbreviations in hospital charts can be overwhelming to someone unfamiliar with medical terminology. When talking with a patient, the nurse should avoid use of medical jargon, acronyms (initials), and abbreviations unless certain they are familiar to the person. For example, Mr. Green is an elderly gentleman who is in the hospital for diagnosis.

> *Nurse:* Mr. Green, we need to cath you for a sterile spec now. The GI series is tomorrow so you will be NPO after midnight.
> *Mr. G.:* Oh? (nurse leaves room)
> *Mr. G. (to wife):* What are they going to do?

Mr. Green had no idea what the nurse had meant. Even within a hospital, each department has its own specific list of initials which may be unfamiliar to the staff on another unit.

Appropriate Timing. Timing can be an important aspect of effective communication. In the clinical setting the patient may be groggy from a pain injection, may have received upsetting news from the family, or may have been told by the physician of a grave diagnosis. The current status should be assessed before communicating with the patient.

Relevance. The message must be relevant to the receiver's interests and concerns if it is to be well received. How does a person respond to a message about astrophysics if the meaning of the term is barely understood? Any communication with patients should center primarily around their concerns, interests, and needs. The personal problems of the nurse and fields of interest unfamiliar to the patient should not be brought into the conversation.

Adaptability. A good communicator is aware of any behavioral cues indicating that the other person does not understand or does not want to follow the current line of communication. A change in mood or a loss of attention may be observed. The communication must be adapted to the individual and to the current situation.

Adaptability includes the ability to phrase the communication in language the receiver can understand. Consider the following situation: Mr. Brown, a construction worker with an eighth-grade education, has been hospitalized for the first time in his life.

> *Nurse:* Mr. Brown, the doctor wants to take some X-rays of your stomach in the morning. Have you ever had these tests before?
> *Mr. B.:* No, but I've had chest X-rays.
> *Nurse:* They will use the same type of X-ray machine, but you will have to drink some white liquid before they start so they can see your stomach on the X-ray. You cannot have anything to eat or drink after midnight tonight or the X-ray pictures won't be good. Do you have any questions?

This message is adapted to the patient and illustrates the necessity of patient assessment. Knowledge of background and general language usage as well as current physical and emotional status facilitates effective communication.

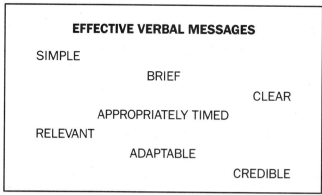

Table 1.1 Effective verbal messages

Credibility. Credibility is extremely important in nursing communication. A good communicator is credible and the message is believable. To be credible, verbal messages must be honest, display knowledge of the subject, reflect confidence, be consistent, and be reliable. If the nurse's communication does not reflect credibility, the patient will not accept what the nurse tries to convey and, consequently, will not be willing to follow directions. The patient's trust is gained through honest, believable communication.

Paralanguage

Paralanguage components are vocal cues other than words, such as the intonation, rate, pitch, and volume associated with the words used. Fluency, vocal patterns, inflection, and dialect that tends to reflect regional or geographic influences are aspects that tend to be built into communication patterns. These are not easily altered and will not be included in the discussion.

Intonation

Intonation can change the entire meaning of words. It is, more or less, the melody of speech. It places emphasis on words or phrases. The following examples illustrate the point:

> The nurse answers a patient's light. As she enters the room she asks, "What can I do for you now?" When the question is repeated, placing the emphasis on a different word each time, the emphasis changes the general meaning of the question. This is exemplified by the following statements:

> I will *not* take that medicine.
> I will not take *that* medicine.

How can they be interpreted? The first seems to convey an unwillingness to take any medicine. The second indicates that a different medicine might be acceptable.

Rate

It is easily observed that people speak at different rates of speed in normal conversations, some slowly and others rapidly. Rapid speech may be as easily understood as slower speech. Rate includes the number and length of pauses. Some newscasters use pauses very effectively, while pauses in another speech may seem awkward and convey uncertainty. The rate of speech is often speeded up with excitement, words tumbling over each other to get out. The status of the other person must be considered in gauging the rate of speech. Older persons with some hearing loss are better able to understand what is said when the rate is slow. Speaking slowly not only makes the words more distinct but gives the person spoken to time to "sort out" what has been said. Patients for whom standard English is not a primary language may benefit from a slower rate of speaking to allow for interpretation.

Pitch

Pitch is determined by the frequency of the sound waves of the voice—the high or low tones. Pitch can be consciously altered within a limited range. A lower pitch is more readily understood by anyone with hearing difficulties. Unconscious changes in pitch may reflect emotions. When excited, voice pitch is often considerably higher.

Volume

Volume is the loudness or softness of the voice. Some people have naturally loud voices that can be heard easily at a distance. Others have very soft voices and can speak loudly only with effort. Everyone varies voice volume to fit the occasion. In a noisy room the tendency is to increase the volume. Voices are muted in situations in which a quiet atmosphere is needed.

Paralanguage can change the meaning of spoken words. It can convey several impressions at the same time. It is important to keep in mind the way words will be decoded with the application of these techniques because, generally speaking, the meanings perceived from spoken words are as dependent on paralanguage and nonverbal components as the actual words.

CHECK IT OUT

Tell a friend what a marvelous time you had at a party. Use a bored monotone while telling the story and interject a few sighs. See if you are believed.

Nonverbal Communication

Communication is not restricted to verbal exchanges. It is often said that actions speak louder than words, that behavior can transmit messages. Nonverbal communication is often called silent communication or body language. Part of a person's nonverbal communication is developed by imitation of others, but a portion of it seems to be instinctive. It can be a conscious behavior. More often than not, however, it is an unconscious reaction to another or an accompaniment of verbal utterances.

Nonverbal messages may be difficult to interpret. The total context of the situation must be considered. Verbal communication can be difficult because of cultural differences. The same holds true of nonverbal communication. Different cultures have different standards or "rules" of nonverbal behavior. In the United States, young people who look an adult straight in the eye are considered open and honest. Spanish cultures consider this disrespectful; in Madrid, young people keep their eyes downcast when talking to an elder. A kiss on the cheek between two men is accepted in most parts of Europe, but it is frowned on in other parts of the world.

The verbal component contributes about one third of the message in face-to-face communication. Nonverbal cues are potent reflections of emotions. A slight sound or almost imperceptible motion can change the meaning of words. Nurses should be very attentive to the patient's nonverbal communication, as the following example illustrates:

Mr. Kemp is a very successful businessman and greatly respected in the community. He has had very few health problems and has never been in a hospital. He was admitted this afternoon for cardiac studies. When the nurse enters his room at bedtime, he is sitting in the chair with a book in his hand, but he is obviously not reading. His shoulders are slumped and his head is bent forward.

Nurse: Mr. Kemp, are you ready to go to sleep?
Mr. K.: No, I think I'll read a bit longer.

Nurse: You seem to be worried about the tests you are having tomorrow.
Mr. K.: (with a forced smile) Nothing that minor is going to bother me.

What would the nurse conclude?
Does his verbal or nonverbal message say more?

Nonverbal behaviors of the nurse are also important. The patients and their families may believe that some facts are kept from them and may watch the health professional very closely for any nonverbal indications of the current status of the patient.

Aspects of nonverbal communication including physical appearance, posture and gait, eye contact, facial expressions, gestures, touch, and body position will be discussed in the following paragraphs.

Physical Appearance

A person's physical appearance influences the reactions of other persons. Fat people are expected to be jolly, and thin persons tense. Skin color, hair length, general appearance, make-up, and jewelry can influence others. Clothes, sometimes said to make the person, can communicate economic status, occupation, and values as well as affect self-image. When a female patient begins to use make-up or a man combs his hair and uses after-shave or cologne, it is often an indication that the patient is on the road to recovery.

Physical appearance can color the perception of a person's message. An unkempt appearance tends to make the words seem less credible. On the other hand, a clean, neat, appropriately dressed individual delivering the same message tends to be more believable. This does not mean to presume that appearance makes a person any more or less truthful, only that appearance influences communication.

Posture and Gait

What can be read about strangers from their walk? Standing straight, head erect, and a bounce in the step indicate self-confidence, while stooped shoulders, a lowered head, and a shuffling step convey low self-esteem. The nurse who stands straight and walks with a purposeful step conveys an air of confidence and competence. Sitting postures are equally expressive, as shown in the previous example of Mr. Kemp.

Eye Contact

Eyes, which are often said to be the mirrors of the soul, are an important aspect of nonverbal communication. Eye movements are not formulated in advance. People are seldom aware of what their eyes are saying but frequently notice what someone else's eyes say.

The amount of eye contact considered acceptable can vary in different cultures. In the United States it is considered important to balance the amount of eye contact during conversations between staring, which is construed as rudeness, and avoiding eye contact, which is interpreted as disinterest. The British, on the other hand, gaze intently at the speaker and expect the same response when speaking.

Eye contact is often avoided when the conversation makes a person feel uncomfortable, while there may be strong eye confrontation during a quarrel. Tension can often be created in others by staring at them. The term "good eye contact" does not necessarily mean that there is a constant mutual gaze between two people.

Facial Expressions

Because faces are so visible and so expressive and the expressions so fleeting, people tend to pay more attention to facial expressions than to other nonverbal behaviors. Some people tend to express feelings readily. It is these persons whose facial expressions tell the most. Others tend to be deadpan. They must be observed closely to detect the subtle nuances that indicate emotions.

The eyebrows are usually very expressive. They may be raised when a person is surprised or puzzled. When drawn together in a frown, they can express displeasure, thoughtfulness, or pain. A sincere smile is considered an expression of happiness. A person may display different emotions at the same time, for example, a slight frown may be accompanied by a faint smile. All cues may be taken together to accurately assess the meaning.

Gestures

Gestures are used for numerous purposes. Hands are used to accentuate, punctuate, and clarify verbal messages. Gestures can be the only means of communication for patients unable to speak.

Persons from different cultures tend to use varying gestures. Italians and Latin Americans tend to use sweeping gestures to punctuate sentences. Caucasian Americans are usually more subdued in use of hands. It has been said that persons who freely use gestures are extroverts. Hiding hands supposedly symbolizes shyness. The tapping of fingers, twisting a ring on the finger, and fidgeting indicate tension. Quiet hands can convey calmness or tension. Some feelings can be determined by noting slight movements of arms or hands in close acquaintances. Gestures must be interpreted in context and related to the individual.

Touch

The importance of touch has received increased attention in the past few years. Touch can communicate warmth, understanding, affection, nurturing, and caring. Some people are instinctive "touchers," while others could be described as "nontouchers." This is not to say that either is right or wrong, simply that people are different. Touching is primarily a spontaneous reaction but may not be a natural response. The use of touch to convey an attitude of caring to patients can be learned and made a part of planned care.

Several factors, including gender, cultural background, and the location and type of touch, influence response to touch. Gender can be a factor. While the average male patient would enjoy a backrub by a female nurse, many would object to the same procedure performed by a male nurse. Cultural background makes a difference. The British tend to be a noncontact group, and Latins are at the other end of the continuum. Scandinavians are in the middle, and Anglo-Saxon

Americans are between the English and the Scandinavians. There are still wide variations within each culture. The location and type of touch are other considerations. The functional professional touch most commonly used in nursing interventions is normally accepted without question, even though it may be in an intimate location. The nurse uses touch, such as holding the patient's hand or touching the arm, to express concern and caring.

Touching is important for all ages. Studies have shown that infants fail to thrive without touch. Elderly persons have a greater need for touch than younger adults since they are more often alone and less mobile. Since several generations seldom live under one roof in today's society, the elderly are deprived of the closeness of grandchildren that former generations enjoyed.

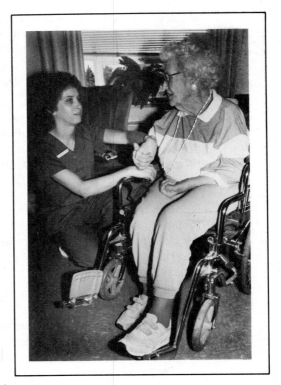

Body Position

Body positions can reveal attitudes. In general, open positions are taken to mean receptiveness, while closed positions indicate withdrawal. However, this does not always hold true. Folded arms may indicate either lack of warmth or a lack of anything better to do with the arms. Crossed legs may be the most comfortable position for the person.

Another aspect of position is the relative position of two people, termed vertical versus lateral. In vertical (or up-and-down) position, the person in the lower position tends to be intimidated. Lateral position, on the other hand, places the communicating parties at equal eye level. When the nurse sits down by the side of the bed, the nurse and the patient are on an equal level. The seated position likewise conveys the message that the nurse has time for the patient. The proximity of the nurse to the patient carries a similar message. The nurse who tends to remain on the other side of the room to communicate expresses an attitude of aloofness, unfriendliness, or fear of contracting the patient's disease.

Some generalizations have been drawn as to the meanings of the various aspects of nonverbal communication. These should not be taken as final answers or definitive interpretations. One action should not be taken out of context in "reading" nonverbal behavior. The message should be interpreted only after assessing the patient and the situation; then, the interpretation must be validated.

CHECK IT OUT

Approach a seated classmate, friend, or family member with a purposeful stride. Remain standing with a firm hand on the shoulder and remind the person that a paper is due, keeping a frown on your face. Try giving the same message to another person while seated. Gently touch an arm and deliver the message with a smile. What difference did the nonverbal communication make?

INFLUENCES ON THE COMMUNICATION PROCESS

Communication does not take place in a vacuum. It is influenced by factors other than the verbal and nonverbal aspects, such as physical setting, space and distance, frame of reference, feedback, interferences, and incongruences in communication.

Physical Setting

The hospital setting can have an impact on nurse-patient communication. Patients not familiar with hospitals can be overwhelmed by the maze of hallways, the noise of the paging system, the unfamiliar medical equipment, the sterile atmosphere, and the profuse use of white. The patient may feel that privacy has been invaded. The nurse must be alert to the verbal and nonverbal aspects of the patient's communication that may indicate that a need for security is taking precedence over current physical needs. The nurse can and should be instrumental in orienting the new patient to the hospital setting and encouraging an expression of needs.

Communication in the health care situation is affected by the specific setting. The atmosphere in an outpatient unit tends to be relaxed. The disorders treated in this area are generally not considered as serious as those treated in other areas. Patients expect to go home the same day. Information is given regarding the procedures that will be followed, discharge instructions are clarified, and any questions that patient may have are discussed just as in other areas in the hospital. Communication in outpatient units, however, is usually somewhat casual, with more socialization, and personnel appear to have more time to talk with patients.

In an intensive-care setting the patient is inundated with stimuli; alarms, lights, phones, and the bustle of the personnel create an atmosphere of tension. Much of the nurse's communication with the patient will be directed toward reassurance. Carefully explaining procedures and equipment often helps relieve fears. For patients who are unable to speak, a system of communication must be developed, whether it is blinking the eyes or moving a toe. Frequent reorientation may be necessary. Telling the patient of pleasant current events helps reduce the sense of isolation from the world. Most patients will not have the energy to talk at length, nor should they be encouraged to do so.

In the general hospital setting, presence of a roommate can be a barrier to communication, especially if one person is much sicker than the other. The nurse can be instrumental in admitting or transferring patients to avoid this difficulty. If the patient is ambulatory or able to be up in a wheelchair, there is the option of going to another area where there is some privacy.

Specific communication techniques explored in later chapters are those applied most frequently in the general hospital setting.

Space and Distance

Proxemics deals with the distance in which a person is comfortable in the environment and in interacting with others. The following four space categories are generally accepted for specified situations:

1. Intimate space (3 to 18 inches). Limited to very close friends.
2. Personal space (18 inches to 4 feet). Suitable for conversations with well-known acquaintances. Usually considered the most effective space for nurse/patient interactions.
3. Social space (4 to 12 feet). Preferred by most for interactions with little-known acquaintances.
4. Public space (beyond 12 feet). Considered preferable for strangers in public places.

There are many variations in these categories related to setting, age and sex of participants, and cultural and ethnic backgrounds. Generalizations must be made cautiously. Each individual has a specific sense of personal space and becomes very uncomfortable or even angry if this space is invaded. The nurse must determine the approximate bounds of each patient's space and respect those boundaries. While one patient may prefer to have the nurse sit next to the bed while talking, another patient might be most uncomfortable and would rather the nurse sit across the room.

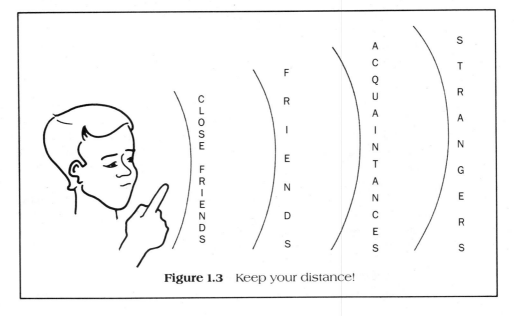

Figure 1.3 Keep your distance!

It is important that a sense of privacy be maintained to as great a degree as possible since patients often experience a loss of privacy. A simple knock on the door before entering a room will go a long way to help maintain this sense of privacy. The nurse should refrain from rearranging personal articles or placing them out of sight without first asking the patient. The hospital room is the patient's current "home" and should be treated with the same respect as if visiting another person's home.

CHECK IT OUT—Space Invasion

Select a person you know well, such as member of your family. Change your normal "nearness" pattern. Keep moving closer and note the reaction. Teenagers are good ones to try this on since they usually express their concerns readily. Just tell them what you were doing after the "invasion."

Frame of Reference

No one is ever isolated at one point in time. Everything that has happened in the past is a part of the present self. Anything that has touched a person's life has left a lasting impression, whether the person was consciously aware of it or not. These background life experiences are part of what is termed frame of reference. Frame of reference embodies culture, religion, family life, socioeconomic status, education, friendships, and all experiences. It includes the individual's current status as well as the past.

The participant's frame of reference can interfere with or enhance communication. When a message is decoded, all of the past as well as the current status enters into the decoding process. The receiver's perception of the message may be quite different from the sender's intention. Effectiveness of communication is enhanced by commonality of experiences. No two persons, not even siblings within a family, have identical frames of reference. Figure 1-4 is an illustration of the frames of reference of participants in a communication interaction. The crosshatched area indicates similarities in backgrounds that will vary with the participants. The more comparable the backgrounds of two people, the more readily they are able to communicate.

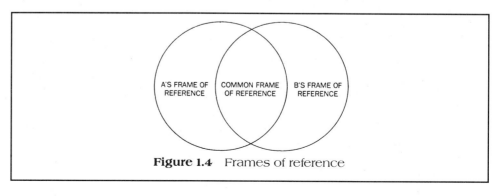

Figure 1.4 Frames of reference

Nurses must communicate with persons of diverse backgrounds and experiences. Cognizance of another person's background affects the manner in which messages are encoded as well as decoded. It is essential for the nurse to try to understand how members of other groups think, feel, and characteristically respond. It is impossible to anticipate the response of every patient. It is possible, however, to learn many details of customary responses of various cultural and ethnic groups and the patient's background. The more background information the nurse has, the greater the ability to communicate effectively.

Feedback

Feedback is sometimes considered a component of the communication process because it is the response of the receiver to the sender's message. It may be linked with listening, since it indicates that the receiver has heard the message. Without feedback the speaker becomes frustrated and feels unaccepted. Feedback is the response given back to the speaker to specify how the message has been interpreted. It enables the sender to determine whether or not the message has been decoded as intended so that it can be rephrased if necessary.

In interpersonal communication, both participants act as senders and receivers, respond to and receive responses, and give feedback to the other. Feedback has an effect on both participants—it keeps communication flowing. If the flow is one-way, communication becomes stagnant and is halted.

Feedback may be verbal or nonverbal, positive or negative. A nod of the head may indicate understanding; a blank stare may show confusion. Feedback may be actions, such as following directions. It may be the exact response anticipated by the sender or the opposite response, or it may consist of diverse verbal and nonverbal responses. Awareness of the other person as an individual can influence the manner in which communication is directed and enhance the response, thus providing more precise feedback. The feedback given should be clear and prompt. It should be in response to a specific message, not a reaction to the speaker. People should listen to themselves when they give feedback and check the effect it has on the other person.

Interferences in Communication

Communication is intended to recreate in the receiver the same message that the sender encoded. Anything that breaks the flow of communication is considered an interference. Possible points of interference are depicted in Figure 1-5. Interference may consist of external factors in the environment or internal factors related to the current status of the receiver. The decoding process is affected by any interference.

External Interferences

Many interferences, such as interruptions, television or stereo blaring, or street noise, occur in everyday communication interactions. These interferences are annoying, but individuals can cope with them. Communication with patients may be rendered ineffective under similar circumstances. External interferences may be in the form of common hospital noises—phones ringing, the intercom blaring, or alarms sounding.

Light may tend to interfere with communication. The level of light in the room may be too low or too bright, or a light may be flashing on a piece of equipment. Glare can be very distracting, especially for older persons. The temperature of the room may interfere with communication. A person is not comfortable when either too hot or too cold. A cluttered room is distracting to many people. Interruptions such as hospital personnel or visitors entering the room can end the communication process. All of these outside interferences can disrupt the transmission and affect the decoding of a message.

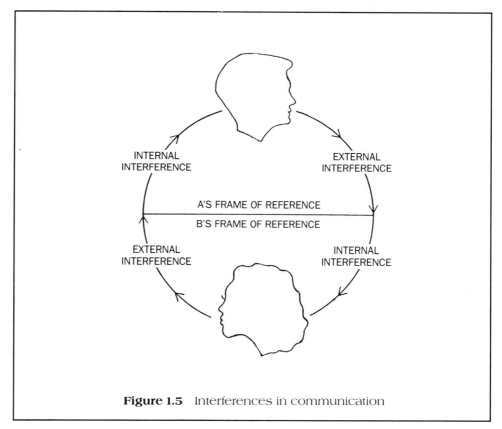

Figure 1.5 Interferences in communication

Internal Interferences

Internal interferences may be related to the physiological or emotional status of the patient. Sensory deficits may be one of the interferences. Hearing deficits may prevent the patient from receiving the message or may result in a misread message. Visual deficits interfere with written and nonverbal messages. Interference in transmission of a message may be linked to past events or to the frame of reference or current physical or emotional status of the receiver. The interference may be what is termed selective inattention, in which the receiver tunes out portions of messages not acceptable at the time. Any internal interference can block or warp reception of the message and have an impact on decoding.

Incongruences in Communication

Verbal and nonverbal communication may not always match. Words may mean one thing and actions or facial expressions another. Miscommunication occurs when a person acts in one way but tells others to act in a different manner. The reaction usually is, "Your actions speak so loudly that I can't hear a word you are saying." In communication, the words may give one message and the nonverbal behavior another. When the nurse asks Mr. Brown how he feels and he replies, "Fine," even though he is slumped down in his chair, avoids eye contact, and speaks in a voice barely above a whisper, what is to be believed, the verbal or nonverbal behavior? This might be the time for the nurse to pull up a chair and chat. The nurse who stands at the door frowning and asks, "May I help you?" does not convey the same message as the one who says the same words while standing at the bedside with a smile.

Any interference in transmission has a definite effect on decoding. The encoding and transmission of a message can alter the effectiveness of communication. The physical setting, paralanguage, and nonverbal components have an impact. Communication is an active, ever-changing, ongoing process. Each component of the communication process as well as factors that influence, enhance, or interfere with communication are constantly changing. Therefore, all aspects of the communication process must continually be reassessed to obtain a valid current appraisal.

THERAPEUTIC COMMUNICATION

All nursing actions should be directed toward meeting patient needs, psychosocial as well as physical. Too often emphasis is on high-visibility actions, the technical procedures. Many patient needs are of an emotional nature. The hospital atmosphere may produce a level of anxiety as well as a feeling of isolation. The patient is often concerned about the illness itself and the financial, work-related, and personal problems it may cause. Communication is the key to meeting the psychosocial needs. The emotional aspects of illness may be difficult for the nurse to cope with, but the patient needs someone who is accepting, understanding, and willing to listen. The more the nurse knows of the patient's background, the better the chance of achieving effective communication.

Therapeutic communication is effective communication. It is the primary aim in nurse-patient interactions. It is a planned type of communication with a purpose. It is a process that follows the nursing process order. Therapeutic communication may have a predetermined goal, or the goal may evolve during a casual interchange.

Therapeutic communication addresses the psychosocial needs of the patient. It is directed toward helping the patient to express feelings, to explore alternatives, and to cope with problems. It lends the emotional support needed. It guides, directs, and structures communication in such a way that the patient can readily verbalize feelings. Application of the facilitative techniques discussed later help to achieve the goals in therapeutic communication.

IN A CAPSULE

Communication is an active, ongoing *process* in which *people exchange messages* using verbal or nonverbal means to effectively convey the intended meaning to the other person. *Communication is learned* by the child during the developmental years influenced primarily by *parental stimulation* and *socioeconomic* and *sociocultural* factors. The *communication process* is comprised of several *components*. An idea serves as the *stimulus* for the sender to *encode* a message to *transmit* to the receiver for *decoding*. The reception of the message is the stimulus for the encoding of a response, and the roles of the sender and receiver are then reversed. To be effective, the *verbal message* should be *simple, brief, clear, appropriately timed, relevant, adapted to the situation,* and *credible*. *Paralanguage*, the intonation, pitch, rate, and volume of speech, can change the perceived meaning of the verbal message.

Nonverbal communication is often more meaningful than verbal. Nonverbal messages include a person's *physical appearance, posture,* and *gait*. *Eye movements* and *eye contact* along with *facial expressions* are prime aspects of nonverbal communication. *Gestures, touch,* and *relative position* may enhance or negatively alter the verbal message. Nonverbal messages must be interpreted cautiously within the total context of the communication interaction.

The *physical setting* has an effect on the communication process. Individuals have *space* and *distance* bounds within which they feel comfortable. An individual's *frame of reference*, that is, all of his or her background experiences, influences each step in the communication process.

Feedback is essential for clarification that the message was decoded as sent. *External or internal interferences* may interrupt the flow of communication. These may be *environmental factors* or may originate within the individual, such as *sensory deficits* and *physical or emotional factors*. *Incongruences* in verbal and nonverbal communication result in a confused message, with the nonverbal aspects often being given the most weight. The nurse can help meet the patient's psychosocial needs through the use of *therapeutic communication*.

DO YOU REMEMBER

- why communication is called a process?
- what constitutes a message?
- how various factors influence language and communication development?
- the essential elements in communication?
- the elements of an effective verbal message?
- what is included in paralanguage?
- the specific nonverbal behaviors discussed?
- what is meant by therapeutic communication?

CAN YOU DESCRIBE

- the stages of language development in infancy and early childhood?
- the cultural differences reflected in what is termed standard and nonstandard speech?
- each of the components in the process of communication?
- the concept of space and distance?
- the impact of the frame of reference on the participants in the communication process?
- the effect of feedback on communication?
- the effect of external interferences on communication?
- the influence of internal interferences on communication?
- how incongruences in communication confuse the interpretation?

ACTION, PLEASE

1. In small groups, spend a few minutes getting acquainted. Determine the special interests and fields of knowledge of the other members of the group.
   a. Draft a volunteer to encode a message to the group using terms that will be unfamiliar. How much of the message did the group understand?
   b. Have the volunteer repeat the message using generally familiar terms. How well was the message understood when it was reworded?
   c. How is this exercise applicable to the nurse-patient communication?

2. Influences on verbal messages. Record a short conversation with a patient or a friend. Note the physical setting, the paralanguage, and the nonverbal behaviors that affected the verbal message. Identify any perceived interferences.
   a. Verbal messages

   _____

   _____

   _____

   _____

   _____

   b. Physical setting

   _____

   _____

   c. Paralanguage

   _____

   _____

   _____

d. Nonverbal behaviors

_____

_____

_____

e. Interferences

_____

_____

_____

What factors, if any, would have made the messages more effective?

_____

_____

_____

3. _What Would You Do?_ You have been assigned to care for Mrs. Carlson, a 58-year-old woman who was admitted with stomach problems. Tests have determined that she has cancer of the stomach. She is in a semiprivate room and the other patient has many visitors. Mrs. Carlson seems very depressed but is reluctant to talk.

a. How would you arrange the environment to promote communication?

_____

_____

_____

b. What nonverbal behavior would be appropriate?

_____

_____

_____

c. What assessments of Mrs. Carlson would you make?

_____

_____

2

Positive Nurse-Patient Relationships Through Communication

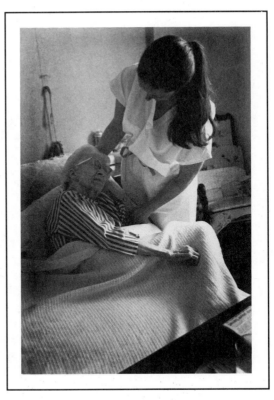

Teach me to feel another's woe, to hide the fault I see. That mercy I to others show, that mercy show to me. **Alexander Pope**

OBJECTIVES

Upon completion of this chapter, the student will be able to:

- identify influences on the continuing development of self-concept.
- relate values clarification to understanding of self.
- note the influence of self-concept on communication.
- discuss ways to improve self-esteem.
- compare defensive reactions and defense mechanisms.
- recall an example of the following defense mechanisms—regression, denial, displacement, and rationalization.
- give reasons for the nurse to communicate with patients.
- describe approaches that help to establish a trusting relationship with a patient.

- contrast empathy and sympathy.
- state ways in which the nurse can communicate empathy.
- define the active listening process.
- list habits and hindrances that interfere with effective listening.
- note behaviors that will improve listening skills.
- discuss factors that are important in building a helping relationship.

GLOSSARY OF TERMS*

Advocate   One who pleads the cause of another.

Defense mechanism   Primarily subconscious response to anxiety that enables the ego to reach compromise solutions to problems.

Denial   Refusal to admit a truth or reality.

Displacement   Substitution of another object as target in expressing feeling against the person or thing causing the unacceptable emotion.

Empathy   The capacity for participation in another person's feelings.

Privileged communication   Confidential information given by the patient to a health care professional pertinent to health history or personal information divulged in the course of care that is unrelated to health care; the recipient is not forced to disclose the information when it is classified as privileged communication.

Rationalization   Justifying one's behavior by stating motives other than the genuine ones.

Regression   A shift toward a lower level of development.

Self-concept   The mental image one has of oneself.

Self-esteem   Relationship of perceived self to desired self; self-respect.

Values clarification   Periodic review of personal value system to determine which principles are currently meaningful and which values are important.

*Definitions applicable to content.

The establishment of a positive relationship between patient and nurse is an important aspect in the effective delivery of total patient care. Nursing is more than the application of proper techniques and procedures in physical care; it is a helping profession in which the nurse communicates a caring attitude and shows concern for the patient. The many technological advances and the computerization of various aspects of health care sometimes seem to reduce the patient to an object. A positive relationship between patient and nurse in which the primary focus is the specific needs of the patient maintains an essential human link. It is the responsibility of the nurse to forge this link, to establish rapport with the patient. This positive relationship can be attained only through communication. To communicate effectively with others, it is necessary to know oneself and be comfortable with this knowledge.

SELF-KNOWLEDGE

Self-Concept

Self-concept is a term frequently heard but often not seriously considered. Self-concept is how persons see themselves—how they think their behaviors are accepted and their idea of who or what they are. It is very difficult for persons to see themselves objectively. A natural tendency is to look outward and observe others rather than to look inward and see the self.

The development of self-concept begins in childhood and is influenced by all significant others. The self-concept tends to act as a self-fulfilling prophecy. A child who is capable but whose efforts are continually criticized will seldom attain his or her potential because of a negative self-concept. On the other hand, a child of average mentality who is praised and encouraged in positive ways to achieve may accomplish far more than is predicted. This can also apply to students. If continually criticized by others, their efforts may subconsciously lessen and they will not accomplish

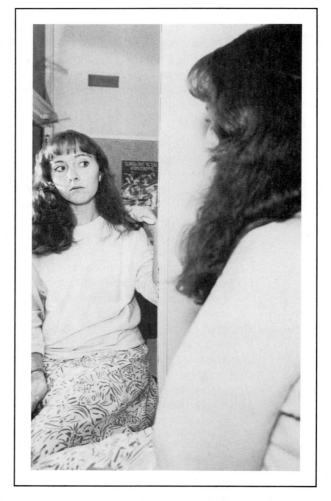

their best. But if they are encouraged and praised, they will see their successes as steps toward their goal. If made to feel worthwhile, a positive attitude toward self results.

The way in which persons picture themselves may be quite different from the way in which others see them. To develop a realistic self-concept they must look at themselves as objectively as possible. Everyone has positive and negative feelings, desires, and behaviors. No one is completely good or bad. To determine self-concept the undesirable traits as well as the positive aspects must be viewed. The opinion one has of oneself is reflected in behavior; a person with a positive self-concept can accept negative feelings or actions and will make an effort to correct any perceived personal faults.

In developing a realistic self-concept, the ever-changing environment must be considered. The world is not static, nor does a person's self-concept remain unchanged. The expectations of others change as individuals change; problems vary with the circumstances. Individual responses must change accordingly or an unrealistic self-concept will develop.

CHECK IT OUT

Below is a list of words that can be used to describe a person. With a small group of friends, have each person select a word to describe self as well as each member of the group. Discuss the results to see how closely the descriptions match.

Friendly	Intelligent	Assertive
Reserved	Slow learner	Bashful
Serious	Caring	Passive
Lighthearted	Distant	Aggressive

Values Clarification

Clarification of values increases self-understanding, thus making self-concept more realistic. To discuss values clarification, it is necessary first to consider the dynamics of value systems. Values are principles or qualities that are believed to be intrinsically desirable, an integral part of the personality. Early in life, individuals develop a value system that is culturally based. Children tend to accept values that are instilled by parents and significant others. However, since value systems are related to life experiences, the development is an active, ongoing process. As the child matures and encounters new situations, the old values may be questioned, with some basic values retained and some altered. Hierarchies are established within the value systems that place some values in a more important position than others. This ranking of values also is subject to change as the situation changes.

Since value systems are dynamic and related to current circumstances, a conscious, periodic review of values can be very meaningful. This review is termed values clarification. The process helps to determine what is most important. It is a method of considering the alternatives available, making a decision regarding the importance of each, and acting on the decision. Values clarification does not mean the establishment of a set of rules, morals, and ethics. It is a close look at the principles that the individual considers most desirable. These values have a key position in choices and become standards that guide actions.

Values clarification is important in choosing a profession because satisfaction in a profession is tied to congruences in professional and personal values. If the values are compatible, there should be no specific conflict in the realm of values. Compassion, competence, and commitment are values in the nursing profession. In nursing there are many ethical dilemmas within the scope of these values— conflicts resulting from the relative values of life itself, freedom from pain, death with dignity, and the patient's right to make decisions. It is never an easy choice.

The understanding and clarification of a value system should increase an individual's acceptance of and respect for value systems of others. A person with a different set of values may be from another culture or simply may not see things the same way. Clarification of one's values does not indicate that these same values are right for others, nor does it imply that these values should be imposed on others.

As values are clarified, understanding of self is increased and a clearer and more realistic self-concept is established. Neither value systems nor self-concept remains static; both change in response to changing circumstances.

Influence of Self-Concept on Communication

Contradictory as it seems, you learn about yourself primarily by communicating with others, and your interpersonal communication is based on your own self-concept. The influence of self-concept on communication is a two-way street. Both persons in a communication interaction encode and decode messages according to their view of self. How persons view themselves has an impact on how others are viewed. If individuals see themselves as open and honest with others, they will judge others by how open they are in their communication. Messages are accepted that confirm a person's opinion of self and ignored or distorted if the message conflicts with this self-concept.

Building Self-Esteem

Self-esteem is closely related to self-concept. It is also dynamic, changing in response to circumstances. Each person has a desired self that exhibits characteristics valued and qualities desired. This desired self may or may not be close to the self as perceived. Individuals constantly evaluate themselves; they look closely at the self they want to be and compare this with the self they see. There may be a discrepancy in the self-concept and the desired self. The comparison of the desired self and the perceived self serves to measure self-esteem. The closer the self-concept is to the desired self, the higher the self-esteem. There is an image of a self that is entirely negative, that is, the kind of person one would never want to be. The self-concept is somewhere between the image perceived as desirable and the negative image. Figure 2-1 represents this concept. At the left is zero self-esteem, at the right, maximum self-esteem. The goal of self-evaluation is to effect changes that bring the self-concept closer to the desired image.

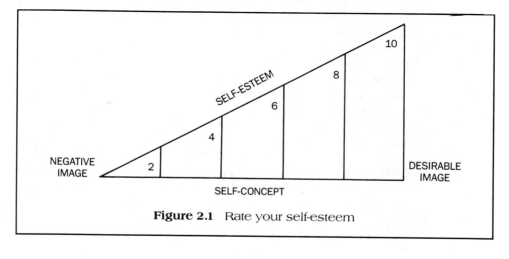

Figure 2.1 Rate your self-esteem

A realistic self-concept is important. If individuals constantly put themselves down and dwell on negative aspects of behavior, self-esteem takes a downward slide. However, the situation is not hopeless. Everyone can change and improve. Control of our lives is possible. The following are ways in which self-concept and/or behaviors can be improved, thus raising self-esteem:

1. Emphasize the positive or good things about yourself. There are no worthless people; some simply think of themselves as worthless.
2. Consider the characteristics of your desired self. Honestly evaluate your behaviors in light of your ideals. Chances are excellent that there are fewer discrepancies than you had previously thought.
3. Choose a characteristic you value and consciously change your behavior to meet this expectation. For example, if you value self-discipline and have always been a procrastinator, set a goal that can be met in a single day and accomplish this goal. Accomplish other daily goals, then progress to longer term goals and strive to meet them. You may be surprised to see the changes in yourself.
4. Stand on your own two feet. You are as capable of making a decision that affects yourself as anyone else.
5. Help others, because in helping others we make ourselves feel better about ourselves.
6. Cultivate relationships that boost your self-confidence. Seek out someone who makes you feel better about yourself and work toward strengthening the bonds of friendship.
7. Above all, don't feel sorry for yourself, thinking you are no good. Look in the mirror and know that you are getting closer to your desired self each day.

Defensive Reactions and Defense Mechanisms

Individuals tend to preserve their self-esteem through the use of defensive reactions and defense mechanisms. Recognizing these behaviors increases understanding of self and others. Defensive reactions and defense mechanisms are responses to anxiety and attempts to protect the ego, to defend the self from perceived threats, and to maintain a high self-esteem. Defense mechanisms are patterns of reactions that take place primarily at the subconscious level. They may be incorporated into a pattern of readily available responses to anxiety-provoking situations. Defense mechanisms enable a person to cope with problems that would be overwhelming otherwise. They serve to protect the self—to keep the ego intact. Defensive reactions differ from defense mechanisms in that defensive reactions take place primarily at the conscious level.

Defensive Reactions

Defensive reactions are used to maintain some control of a situation. These behaviors reflect emotional states that may be triggered by a specific topic introduced in the conversation or may result from the accumulation of irritations. Patients find themselves in a vulnerable position when they enter a hospital, being told what to do and when to do it, being asked personal questions by total strangers, and giving up their privacy. Students may find themselves in a similar situation, especially if they are returning to the classroom after a period of independent living. Defensive strategies are used in an attempt to maintain control. They are responses to the circumstances rather than responses aimed toward the hospital personnel and should not be construed as a personal attack.

Anger or hostility is a frequent response to a perceived threat. A patient may respond with anger when asked a question regarding personal habits such as drinking, especially if this is a problem. Being aware that this is a defensive reaction will give the nurse a better understanding of the behavior and a realization that the anger is not a personal attack.

Changing the subject is another frequently used defensive reaction. This often occurs in nurse-patient communication, and it is not always the patient who changes the subject. Nurses may suddenly turn the conversation to the current procedure or remember something that necessitates leaving the room when the patient introduces a topic such as impending death if the nurse is not comfortable discussing the subject.

Jokes and trivial remarks may be used as defensive behaviors. Making a joke out of a situation tends to convey the idea that it does not really matter. An elderly gentleman who had been a very successful businessman told jokes constantly in an apparent attempt to avoid the serious conversations he had formerly enjoyed but was no longer able to maintain as a result of some loss of memory resulting from a stroke.

Nonverbal reactions may be defensive responses. The body responds physiologically to emotional states. Muscles may tense and the body may tend to stiffen when an unpleasant subject is introduced. Vocal tones and paralanguage may be involved in defensive reactions. The voice may rise and become louder in an emotionally upsetting situation. Being aware of what may happen within helps to interpret what might be happening in others. However, nonverbal cues should be interpreted with caution. Feedback is essential to ensure the accuracy of interpretation.

Defense Mechanisms

Identification of defense mechanisms can give a better understanding of patient behaviors. The defense mechanisms of regression, denial, displacement, and rationalization, along with examples of each, are discussed in the following paragraphs. These are only a few of the more common defense mechanisms that tend to affect nurse-patient communication in the general clinical setting.

Regression is the return to an earlier level of functioning in an attempt to escape a current conflict. This may be seen in children who start bed-wetting long after they have been trained. The arrival of a new baby in the family will sometimes trigger this behavior. It can be seen in hospitalized persons who tend to become completely dependent on the staff for care even though they are capable of doing many things for themselves. For example, a nurse was surprised to see a 12-year-old boy who had been hospitalized following a bicycle accident sucking his thumb.

Denial is the refusal to admit that a situation exists. It is a defense mechanism that is not completely subconscious. However, this does not imply that the person chooses not to be aware of unpleasant realities, but that these realities cannot be faced at the present time. Denial may be carried out in fantasy and daydreaming, where the real world is blocked out even though the person knows the fantasy is not real. Denial is often seen in patients who have just been told they have a serious illness. It is also a stage in the grieving process, as illustrated by the following examples:

> The doctor told Mrs. Phipps on his morning rounds that her biopsy indicated a malignancy. When her husband visited her that evening, she told him that the doctor had not been in so she did not know the results of the biopsy.
> Mr. Hornsby, who recently had a heart attack, refused to stay in bed because he said there was nothing wrong with him.

Displacement is one of the better known mechanisms, even though the term may not be frequently used. A substitute is found as the target for release of emotions against the original person or "thing" causing the anxiety-provoking situation. It is important that nurses be aware of this defense mechanism since patients often lash out at nurses simply because they are there. Out of frustration they are finding someone on whom to vent their emotions. It is not a personal attack, as shown in the following example:

> You are giving Mrs. Murphy her bath when she starts telling you that you are a horrible nurse and not taking good care of her. Though not sure of the reason for the tirade, you continue to care for her. As the morning progresses, you find out that a neighbor has informed her of her husband's infidelity while she is in the hospital.

Rationalization is another frequently used mechanism. Plausible reasons are given as explanations for problems or behavior. This is similar to making excuses. There is always a small element of truth, but this is enlarged to justify a behavior by stating other motives for the genuine one.

> Mrs. Carson cancelled a dental appointment because her car had a flat tire. The car did have a flat tire but a neighbor offered to take her. The full truth was she hated going to the dentist.
> A student who failed a nursing exam told a friend that visitors the previous night had kept him from studying adequately.

PURPOSES OF NURSE-PATIENT COMMUNICATION

Understanding self and others promotes communication. Through effective communication rapport is established with patients. Just as communication is basic to all human relationships, it is fundamental in nurse-patient relationships. It is said that the primary reasons patients list for communicating with nurses are to obtain information and for socialization. Nurses communicate with patients for these reasons, but there are other reasons as well. Nurses initiate communication with patients to establish a basis for care and to determine and seek to meet basic needs of patients.

Explore Feelings

Only after the nurse has established rapport can the patient be encouraged to explore feelings. This is therapeutic communication, an important aspect of nurse-patient communication. Student nurses may find this area difficult. Any illness is accompanied by fears, and illness tends to magnify other feelings. Many patients, especially men, are reluctant to admit that they are afraid of anything. If the nurse can, through the use of effective communication techniques, enable the patient to talk about these fears, this will hopefully reduce anxiety. Frequently the fears are unfounded and a simple explanation is all that is necessary. At other times the fears are well-founded, but having someone to talk with serves as a relief value.

Obtaining and Giving Information

The nurse must obtain information from patients in order to determine their current physical and emotional status. Patients are sometimes irritated with all of the questions asked, but it is only with this information that the nurse can make an accurate assessment and plan nursing care. The nurse gives information to the patient throughout the hospital stay: orienting the patient to the hospital routines, explaining procedures and tests, clarifying the physicians' instructions, teaching about the disease, demonstrating procedures, giving discharge instructions, and answering any other questions the patient might have.

Socialization

Socialization is a nursing function, though not a primary one. Patients admitted to the hospital are suddenly cut off from their usual friends and experience loneliness, especially elderly persons. General conversation with patients is important, even if it only consists of chatting about the weather or about their families. A nurse can learn a lot about the patient by listening and can often pinpoint worries. Nurses should not spend 8 hours a day simply talking with their patients, but each time the nurse goes in a room to carry out a procedure, communication can be encouraged. Time can also be scheduled to sit and talk with the patient.

TRUST IN NURSE-PATIENT RELATIONSHIPS

Through communication the nurse is able to establish a trusting relationship with the patient. Trust is assured reliance on the abilities or strength of someone or something. Trust gives a feeling that there are some people in the world who care and are friendly, who can be relied on without question, and who are available to help when needed. This is found in all successful interpersonal relationships. People must trust others in many situations in order to function in this society.

Creating Trust

Patients feel very vulnerable when entering the hospital, where much of their physical care must be entrusted to others. Only when patients feel that they can trust the personnel caring for them can they be comfortable in the hospital environment. This trust is created primarily through communication.

It may be very difficult for a patient who has had an unhappy experience related to hospitalization to trust the personnel. The nurse must prove to the patient that he or she is trustworthy. Often the small details, such as returning to the room when promised, answering questions honestly, or securing the extra pillow requested, can establish trust. Establishing trust takes time; very few people will trust someone on a first encounter.

Privileged Communication

An important aspect of trust is the assurance that the nurse will hold in confidence any personal information not related to health care. Maintaining the confidence of the patient dates back to the Nightingale pledge and is part of the nurses' code of ethics. Nurses, as other professionals, are recipients of privileged information and of facts and feelings that are sometimes very personal and private.

The caring attitude that the nurse ideally conveys provides a secure environment for the patient. Patients thus feel safe in confiding in the nurse and presume that the shared facts or feelings will be held in confidence. Often the nurse is the only person with whom the patient can communicate. The professional attitude of the nurse conveys the idea that private information will not be divulged, but verbal reinforcement strengthens the trusting relationship. Privileged information will be discussed further in a later chapter.

Importance of Honesty

Honesty is an integral part of trust. When a patient asks a question that the nurse cannot answer, this should be acknowledged and an attempt made to obtain the information requested. Evading questions or giving inaccurate answers is not an honest approach. If the nurse will be taking care of the patient for only a short time, the patient must be made aware of the fact. This is important for the student nurse who is in the clinical setting for limited periods to remember. If the time frame is made known from the beginning, the patient will not feel abandoned.

Some situations involving honesty might arise that place the nurse in a difficult position. When the patient asks the nurse about the attending physician, even though the nurse is not certain of the physician's competency, the question cannot be ignored. The nurse faces being dishonest with the patient in upholding the physician and faces slander in giving the patient an honest opinion. There is no easy solution to this dilemma. The nurse must be honest in any answers but must also accept responsibility for the reply. The solution may be for the nurse to say, "I am not familiar with some of the doctors in this hospital," which may be entirely true.

Mutual Trust

Trust should never be one-sided. Each person must trust the other for a relationship to be established. Trust is related to the aims and goals of each person. If those of the nurse are congruent with those of the patient, a mutual trust can be established. This mutual trust is sustained by honesty on both sides, but it does not mean that both parties must reveal all facts that the other person requests. For example, if the physician has informed a patient of the diagnosis, it is the responsibility of the nurse to discuss the condition and methods of caring for it. However, if the nurse is not sure whether or not the physician has informed the patient of the diagnosis, the nurse must first find out what information the doctor has given the patient. Remember that either participant in a relationship of mutual trust has the right to refuse to answer a question. This does not negate the mutual trusting relationship but allows both parties to make decisions regarding the facts or feelings they choose to share.

EMPATHIC COMPONENTS IN NURSE-PATIENT RELATIONSHIPS

Empathy is the capacity to understand another's feelings. It is a type of intellectual role playing, an attempt to experience another person's feelings as if they were one's own—to understand how the person feels, reacts, and thinks, and to understand the other person's life, problems, values, and meanings. Empathy involves being sensitive to but not a part of the other person's feelings and to the changes in these feelings. It revolves around active listening, careful observation, and understanding.

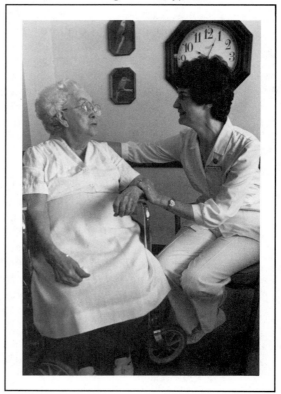

Importance of Objectivity

Objectivity as related to the expression of empathy requires the maintenance of self-identity while being sensitive to the feelings of another. Objectivity is essential to prevent the nurse's own values and feelings from coloring the perception of the patient's problems and feelings. A person can become absorbed in the characters in a book or movie to the extent of being "at one" with them but resume self-identity at the conclusion. This is how empathizing with patients should be. Objective awareness of the patient's world leads to better understanding of their behavior but should not be carried over into the nurse's life. Empathy reflects objectivity and reduces the personal risks of becoming too involved.

Empathy Contrasted with Sympathy

Sympathy differs from empathy in that the sympathetic nurse assumes the feelings of the patient, losing self-identity. Sympathy involves sorrow or pity. Subjective assessments are made and an inaccurate perception of true feelings results. Nurses who allow themselves to feel sorry for the patient will not only make the patient feel uncomfortable but will also put themselves at risk of rapid emotional burnout as patient problems are assumed as their own.

Empathy focuses on the patient with the problem, not on the listener, as sympathy tends to do. Empathy is sharing of feelings rather than expression of a feeling in response to the situation. Empathy is seeing the world through another person's eyes rather than weeping at the plight of another. The sympathetic nurse expresses condolence, while the empathic nurse offers understanding. This is not meant to negate the importance of expressions of sympathy. Sympathy is a specific expression of concern and caring. Sympathy can help as an offer to share problems at a time when they cannot be met alone; but, in the long run, sympathy can make others less able to solve their own problems.

Communicating Empathy

Nurses frequently do not see themselves as expressing empathy, but patients usually see nurses as empathic persons. How is this attitude communicated? Active listening is an important aspect of expressing empathy, concentrating on the patient's verbal and nonverbal messages. Open-ended questioning should be utilized to encourage patients to communicate feelings and concerns. Listening carefully and objectively is essential to an accurate assessment of the status of the patient. After listening carefully, the nurse should take time to absorb what has been said before making a response. Any verbal response should be brief. The communication of empathy is quickly lost in a barrage of words. Responses, both verbal and nonverbal, should reflect the same general feeling as that expressed by the patient. Empathy is more readily expressed by the nurse and perceived by the patient when the two have similar background experiences. A mother with a critically ill child may feel that a nurse who has had a similar experience is more able to appreciate her feelings than the nurse without children.

Communicating empathy can be a learned behavior. The importance of active listening, time to think about the material before replying, and brief verbal responses that reflect the patient's feelings have been noted as important in communicating empathy. Empathic responses tend toward voicing understanding of expressed or implied feelings, for example:

> *Patient:* This new treatment means another week in the hospital.
> *Nurse:* You sound as if you miss your family.

The nurse is attempting to "walk in the shoes" of the patient. This type of response often begins, "You look . . . ," "You sound . . . ," or "It's important to you . . ." It has been suggested that nonverbal behavior plays a larger role than verbal responses in communicating empathy. Eye contact, intonation, facial expressions, and touch often can convey more than words.

CHECK IT OUT

In small groups, consider the following patient statements. Discuss empathic and nonempathic responses to determine the response that would be most natural for the nurse and most supportive for the patient.

I am so disappointed because I have to come back to the hospital for more chemotherapy.

I have been postponing this surgery for 6 months.

I don't think I'll ever be able to walk again after this surgery.

My baby probably won't remember me if I have to stay in this place another week.

My husband hasn't been here to see me for 2 days.

LISTENING BEHAVIORS TO PROMOTE EFFECTIVE COMMUNICATION

It is estimated that about 70% of an adult's waking hours are spent in communication. This includes reading, writing, speaking, and listening. Of this time, over half is spent in listening or, more accurately, hearing. Hearing and listening are not the same. Hearing is the reception of sound waves by the ear, which stimulates the auditory nerves, resulting in sounds being perceived. Listening involves hearing with thoughtful attention.

The average college student retains only about 20% to 25% of the material presented in class. This percentage might be increased by improving the ability to listen. Effective listening skills can be profitable in many ways. Listening can be a shortcut to knowledge since it is faster than reading, especially if several sources must be sought to find the answer. It can improve grades as well as reduce study time. It can improve interpersonal relations and can improve nursing practice in that patients will respond more positively to communication efforts resulting in greater accuracy of assessments.

Active Listening Process

Although it may seem that listening is a passive process in which information is received from another person, active listening requires energy and concentration. Active listening involves not only hearing the spoken words, but noting the nonverbal behaviors. Once the words have been received, they must be organized and interpreted by the listener. Listening demands concentration and the ability to ignore distractions, both external and internal. People can become so involved in personal thoughts that they hear only a part of what is said.

Active listening requires responses on the part of the listener. Most of these responses should be nonverbal or short verbal responses to acknowledge hearing the message, but there should be a response. It is most discouraging to try to talk to someone who sits passively without ever changing his or her facial expression or visibly moving a muscle. Body position—leaning forward in the chair, maintaining good eye contact, and assuming an open posture to convey the idea of an open door—can portray a listening attitude. Short responses, or even nodding the head, can indicate to the speaker that the listener is absorbing what is being said.

Active listening can be for the primary purpose of obtaining information. This is the type of listening students do in the classroom. They make a deliberate attempt to hear the information, organize it, and recall it at a later time. Listening may involve an empathic element in that the goal is to understand what is being communicated from a different point of view—listening as though in the other person's place. It involves full and active attention, an integration of emotional and mental inputs in an attempt to understand the current status of the communicator, noting the nonverbal behaviors as closely as the words spoken. It involves responding to the person as an individual. This type of active listening is one method of communicating empathy.

Ineffective Listening Habits

Listening habits can hinder or facilitate the process. Habits are more readily developed than broken, but it is possible to change them. To successfully break a habit, it is necessary to be aware of the behavior. Some common listening habits that interfere with effective listening include those discussed in the following paragraphs.

Faking Attention

Students may fake attention in class. This is a habit that may be traced to early years in school when a child is disciplined for not being attentive. It can carry over to social situations or, more seriously, to situations in the health care delivery system. The nurse may miss important information about the patient's condition by not paying complete attention to what is being said. This habit can be changed if the

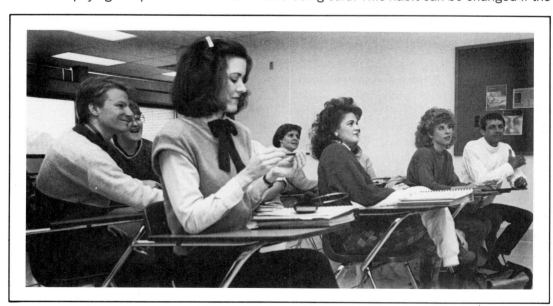

nurse becomes aware of times when attention is faked and attempts to determine the cause. In the clinical setting this may be when asking routine questions. Becoming aware of this problem and being motivated to change are usually sufficient.

Concentrating on Details

Too much attention to details can interfere with effective listening. A student in the classroom may be listening so hard for facts and taking such copious notes that the general idea of the lecture is missed. In communication the nonverbal behaviors and emotions perceived can be as indicative as the facts related. This is especially important in nurse-patient relationships, since patients may be reluctant to verbalize feelings to a person with whom they are not well acquainted. The facts must be taken into account, but the nonverbal accompaniments must also be considered in the overall interpretation. Overcoming the habit of concentrating only on details will require effort and concentration on the part of the listener.

Tuning Out

Sometimes people tune out when the material being discussed is not very interesting or is believed to be too difficult. This problem has been referred to as the "Sesame Street syndrome." Granted, there may be times when the person does not understand or want to know more about the topic being discussed, but the topic can be further explored when there is time and may prove to be more interesting or easier to understand than the person realized. This increases the general knowledge and may make the individual a better listener as well as a more adept conversationalist. If tuning out is a problem, the listener should listen carefully and ask the speaker to make additional explanations if in an appropriate situation such as a small group.

Reacting to the Speaker

The listener may react to the speaker rather than to the words. More attention may be paid to the speaker's clothes or regional accent or to the grammatical structures of the speech than to the context of the message. These things should not distract from listening to what the person is saying. This can occur in the clinical setting where there may be, for example, a gross deformity or an unsightly skin condition. Viewing every speaker as clad in a long black robe may solve this problem.

There are times when emotions take over and the individual reacts emotionally to a word or phrase used by the speaker, closing his or her ears to the remainder of the communication. The response may be one of anger or sadness. Thoughts turn inward and the message is missed. This type of response may be difficult to overcome. Concentration on the speaker's words is the key but will require practice.

Hindrances to Listening

The poor listening habits discussed in the preceding paragraphs are hindrances to effective listening, but other factors also affect the ability to listen. People are frequently selective listeners, hearing only what they want to hear. Children are a prime example of selective listening. They hear parents tell them that the ice cream is ready but fail to hear that they should wash their hands before coming to the table. Emotions can block parts of a conversation that would be painful. Some specific hindrances to listening are noted in the following paragraphs.

Physical and Emotional Factors

Current physical and emotional status may be a factor in the ability to absorb what is heard at a particular time. Emotional factors may range from boredom to anxiety; physical factors include headaches, lack of sleep, and acute pain. Individuals should be aware of their physical and emotional status and reinforce information at a later time if not up to par. In communicating with patients, their current physical and emotional status must be carefully assessed.

Sensory Dysfunctions

With sensory dysfunctions the brain does not receive the stimuli necessary for organization and interpretation, even though the nonverbal cues may be a part of the input received. If there is a hearing impairment, listening will be more difficult. On the other hand, visual impairments will limit the nonverbal cues that enhance a more valid interpretation in the listening process. Checking for sensory dysfunctions should be a part of communication assessment. They may necessitate some adjustments to compensate for loss of input.

Distractions

Distractions can be a major hindrance to listening. Environmental distractions can be more or less controlled—turning off the television, closing the door, or asking the other person to speak louder. Internal distractions are not as easily controlled. It may be difficult for the student to concentrate on what the patient in the clinical setting is saying when there is a possibility that the instructor may enter the room. Distractions also apply to the patient's ability to listen. There is no one solution to removing these internal distractions. This must be resolved on an individual basis.

Lack of Concentration

Failure to concentrate on what the speaker is saying may be a type of internal distraction, a poor listening habit, a physical factor such as a headache, or an environmental factor such as room temperature. The ability to concentrate can be a learned behavior. It requires a conscious effort and rigid self-discipline for some people to develop, while it seems to be a natural response for others.

Importance of Feedback

Feedback is an important aspect of listening, and listeners have a responsibility to give the speaker feedback. Feedback may be verbal, nonverbal, or both. As discussed before, nonverbal communication is often more believable than verbal. However, verbal feedback is also important to the speaker and to the listener. Listeners who are allowed to give feedback and to ask questions during the discourse will retain more of the material than those who are not allowed to give feedback. Any feedback should be directed toward the message rather than the speaker and should pertain to specific points that the speaker has made. If the feedback is made promptly, it tends to be less confusing to the speaker. In one-to-one communication this is readily accomplished since there is an ongoing exchange between the individuals. It is more difficult in a group situation, even though small groups lend themselves well to open discussion. Listening and feedback are hallmarks of effective communication.

Developing Effective Listening Skills

Although many people are not good listeners, good listening habits can be learned and are worth the time and effort required. Some specific suggestions to improve listening skills are listed below:

1. Listen with preparation. Be prepared physically and mentally to listen. Listening requires energy and concentration. If you are under par physically or emotionally, your attention span is greatly reduced.
2. Listen quietly.
3. Listen to content. Hear what the speaker is saying without evaluating appearance or delivery.
4. Pay attention to the nonverbal components of the message. What does the speaker's body language tell you? Does the paralanguage color the message? What is not said? Sometimes topics avoided can be indicative.
5. Listen actively from the beginning. Sometimes listeners wait until a word or phrase catches their attention, but they may have missed important facts leading up to it.
6. Listen to all that the speaker has to say before making an interpretation of the message.
7. Listen courteously. Do not interrupt unnecessarily, try to embarrass the speaker, or attempt to get the speaker off the subject.
8. Listen flexibly. Be flexible and willing to entertain new ideas even though they may not agree with your convictions.
9. Listen attentively. Avoid distractions and poor listening habits discussed previously.
10. Concentrate. This is *the* most important aspect of good, active listening. To concentrate more effectively:
    a. Monitor your listening to make certain your thoughts are not wandering and you are keeping an open mind.
    b. Listen for the main ideas and the general context of the message.
    c. Suspend any interpretation of the message until it is completed, since this will influence your reaction to the remainder of what is being said.
    d. Periodically mentally review what has been said.
    e. Try to view the subject from the speaker's viewpoint.
    f. Utilize the difference in speech rate and thought rate to concentrate on the message.

This last point is a concept deserving special attention. The average person speaks at a rate of 125 to 175 words per minute. If thoughts could be measured, our mental processing ability would lie somewhere between 500 and 1000 words per minute. What our minds do with this lag can be the difference between a good and a poor listener. Too often, our minds will wander to past or anticipated events. By concentrating on the speaker's message, this time lag can be used to review what has been said, to organize the facts given, and to concentrate on the meaning of the message.

BUILDING A HELPING RELATIONSHIP

The preceding discussion covers aspects essential to the establishment of a helping relationship. The importance of active listening cannot be overemphasized. It is the key that opens the door. The role of the nurse is, indeed, a helping role. The physical care administered to the patient is often seen as the primary role of the nurse, but the psychosocial support given by the nurse is equally important. This embodies a helping, empathic relationship that can be a therapeutic adjunct to physical administrations of care.

Acceptance

One of the primary facets in a helping relationship is acceptance of the other person as an individual. The acceptance of others follows self-acceptance, a consequence of high self-esteem. To accept others means to take them at face value, to adopt a nonjudgmental attitude. The nurse may not agree with patients' beliefs and values but can accept them as individuals. The nurse communicates this attitude by accepting remarks, complaints, or criticisms without expressing opinions or imposing conditions. The patient then feels safe and nondefensive, able to cooperate more fully in care.

Sincerity

The nurse must display sincerity, or genuineness, to build a relationship that will be helpful to the patient. Facades are always transparent. The sincere person is comfortable with self and can therefore interact with others on the other person's terms. One aspect of sincerity is consistency or congruence. The nurse's verbal and nonverbal behavior must be congruent and must convince the patient that the words are spoken with sincerity. Sincerity is conveyed by spontaneous expression. An outgrowth of sincerity is trustworthiness or credibility, which is an essential ingredient of any relationship. The patient will trust and believe the nurse who is thought to be sincere.

Respect

Respect may be an appreciation of the "separateness" of another person and of the ways in which the other person is unique. Respect is paramount in building a helping relationship. It is a positive regard for another and is communicated through actions as much as through words. It involves a commitment on the part of the nurse to work with the patient, maintaining a nonjudgmental attitude. Respect indicates an understanding of how the other person feels and communicates interest.

Caring

Caring is another essential in a helping relationship. It involves a feeling of interest in and concern for another, a regard stemming from esteem. Caring may be expressed as warmth communicated through tone of voice, eye contact, facial expression, or touch. This caring attitude or warmth is sometimes nebulously termed a "good bedside manner" and can be as important as the technical competence of the nurse in therapeutic effectiveness. Caring is an attribute that must come from within.

Patient Advocacy

The nurse-patient relatinship is strengthened through the role of the nurse as patient advocate. An advocate defends the cause of another. As a patient advocate the nurse helps patients solve problems encountered in health care situations that they are unable to solve alone. The advocate either seeks a solution or tells the patient how to find a solution to the problem. The patient is helped to make decisions and is supported in any decisions made. The advocate makes certain that the patient knows what to rightfully expect from the health care system.

Listening and communication skills are essential to the role of patient advocate. For example, if the nurse realizes that the patient is not aware of the risks involved in a procedure that is scheduled, the physician should be notified to clarify this to the patient. Signed consent forms are not considered valid if the patient does not understand the risks involved. Awareness that the nurse is concerned about all aspects of their welfare increases the confidence of patients and promotes a positive nurse-patient relationship.

The nurse builds and maintains a helping relationship that conveys acceptance, sincerity, respect, and caring and is further strengthened by the nurse assuming the role of patient advocate. The use of facilitative techniques that promote therapeutic communication will be explored in the next chapter.

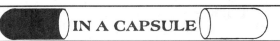

IN A CAPSULE

Knowing yourself enhances communication and relationships with others. A realistic *self-concept* is developed through an objective assessment of positive and negative aspects of behavior. Self-concept does not remain static but changes with maturity and in response to environment. *Values clarification* increases self-knowledge since it requires a conscious consideration of principles or qualities most highly valued, thus clarifying positions in choosing alternatives. Communication is influenced by *self-concept* in the general approach to others used by an individual. *Self-esteem* is a measure of how we perceive ourselves as compared to how we desire to be.

Self-esteem can be increased as behaviors are consciously altered to meet desired standards.

Individuals may use *defensive responses* such as anger in an attempt to maintain control of a situation. *Defense mechanisms* are primarily subconscious responses used to protect the ego and preserve self-esteem. The *nurse* should be perceptive of *patient* reactions when *communicating for various reasons*, most aimed toward building a relationship.

Honesty is essential to create *trust in a nurse-patient relationship.* Assurance that holding any *privileged information* in confidence strengthens the trust. The nurse communicates *empathy* by listening carefully and determining objectively the patient's viewpoint. *Active listening* can be one of the most effective communication tools a nurse employs. It requires concentration and meaningful feedback. Nurses must be aware of any hindrances to listening in the environment, in the patient, and in themselves. A *helping relationship* can be established by incorporating all of the above into patient care plus exhibiting *acceptance*, *sincerity*, *respect*, and a *caring* attitude. This relationship is further strengthened by the *patient advocate* role of the nurse.

DO YOU REMEMBER

- factors relating to the development of a realistic self-concept?
- the relationship of values clarification to self-concept?
- the purpose of defensive reactions?
- the purpose of defense mechanisms?
- why nurses communicate with patients?
- what is meant by privileged communication?
- the difference in empathy and sympathy?
- the ineffective listening habits discussed?
- some hindrances to listening?
- facets in a helping relationship?
- what is meant by patient advocate?

CAN YOU DESCRIBE

- the effect of self-concept on communication?
- ways to improve your self-esteem?
- how a nurse can create mutual trust with a patient?
- the manner in which nurses communicate empathy?
- the process of active listening?
- specific ways in which you can improve your listening skills?

ACTION, PLEASE

1. Self-concept just for you. This is not a group activity but a suggestion to help you increase your self-esteem. Make a chart similar to the one below. List the qualities you most admire in the first column. Honestly assess yourself regarding these characteristics. Set short- and long-term goals to help you acquire any quality that you consider desirable. Note dates when you feel the goal is met. Assess changes you see in yourself.

Desired qualities	Perceived qualities	Goals (short-term, long-term)	Dates goals met	Progress toward desired goals
Honesty	Honest	No problem		
Sociability	Difficulty meeting new people	Talk with six classmates in one day;	9/16	11/18 Talking with others becoming easier
		establish a relationship with two classmates	11/6	

After 5 or 6 months, take another careful look at yourself. Do you feel any closer to you desired self? The closer you get, the higher your self-esteem.

2. Defense mechanisms. After studying the defense mechanisms discussed in the chapter, recall a situation in the past few weeks in which you, or someone with whom you have had contact, used one of these defense mechanisms. Be prepared to discuss it in class.

Defense mechanisms noted _____

Situation and background _____

_____

_____

3. *A Look At Listening*. You have been assigned to care for 72-year-old Mrs. Bullington. The head nurse has asked you to explain to her the tests that are scheduled for tomorrow. You also need information regarding her past and current health status to plan her care.

    a. What assessments will you make to determine her ability to listen to your explanations?

_____

_____

    b. What specific behaviors will convey to her that you are listening to her?

_____

_____

_____

3

Promoting Effective Communication

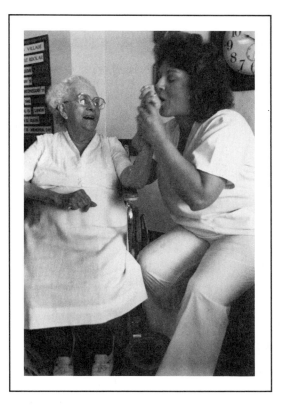

To get full value of a joy, you must have somebody to share it with.
Mark Twain

OBJECTIVES

Upon completion of this chapter, the student will be able to:

- describe ways in which the nurse can arrange an environment conducive to communication.
- discuss background factors of the patient that influence communication.
- assess the physiological and emotional status of patients as related to communication.
- state the importance of active listening in communication.
- discuss the significance of following through on cues.
- note the impact of prejudice and value judgments on communication.
- state purposes of facilitative techniques in communication.
- give examples of the following facilita-

tive techniques:
    Open-ended questions and statements
    Validating
    Acknowledging feelings
    Reassuring
- explain four methods of clarifying a message.
- note the function of silence as a facilitative technique.
- give an example of the following specific blocks to communication:
    Closed-ended questions
    Clichés
    False reassurance
    Defending
    Challenging
    Changing the subject
- list detrimental results of each type of judgmental response.
- list appropriate responses of the nurse to patient blocks in communication.
- define neutral responses.
- discuss the use of humor in communication.
- note areas considered inappropriate in nurse-patient interactions.

GLOSSARY OF TERMS*

Belittle   To cause a person or situation to seem less.

Block   In communication, a response that tends to minimize feedback and prevent further communication.

Clarify   To make clear or understandable.

Facilitate   To make easier.

Judgmental response   Expression of a personal opinion reflecting a judgment of the situation.

Open-ended   Designed to permit spontaneous and unguided responses.

Paraphrase   A restatement giving the meaning in a different form.

Prejudice   An opinion adverse to anything without just grounds or before sufficient knowledge.

Reflect   To give back or repeat a message.

Stereotype   A standardized mental picture of a group that ignores individual differences.

Validate   Confirm or remove doubt regarding the meaning of a message.

Value judgment   Judgment of another person or a situation according to personal standards.

*Definitions applicable to content.

Encouraging the expression of feelings and facts is imperative in effective, therapeutic communication. In everyday interactions, people prefer talking with someone who will hear their personal stories without interrupting to tell theirs and who will express interest by asking questions. This chapter presents methods for nurses to encourage patients to communicate openly. It also explores ways in which communication may be blocked.

GENERAL INFLUENCES ON THE COMMUNICATION PROCESS

Various factors contribute to the general atmosphere or setting of nurse-patient interactions. The communication atmosphere may be considered the total of all variables in communication. This includes the frame of reference of both participants, the rapport between patient and nurse, the readiness to communicate, the status of the patient, the general approach of the nurse, and the setting or immediate environment.

Effect of Environment on Communication

The environmental setting can have a positive or a negative impact on communication. There are some areas, such as general setting, noise, light, interruptions, and time of day, over which the nurse has some control in setting the stage for a communication interaction.

General Setting

The general setting of the room has an effect on communication. If a person is not physically comfortable, it is difficult to keep attuned to the conversation. A room that is too warm or too cool is not comfortable. Lack of adequate ventilation, even when the room is at an acceptable temperature, causes a room to be stuffy and uncomfortable. The temperature can be easily adjusted by the nurse, but the patient's wishes must be considered since some patients, especially elderly ones, prefer a warmer room.

A cheerful, attractive room is considered conducive to communication, and a cluttered room distracting. However, moving the patient's personal items out of sight may be more distracting to them. A sense of privacy is necessary for effective communication. This may be difficult in a semiprivate room, but the nurse can close the curtain, talk in a quiet voice, and face the patient to achieve some privacy. The nurse's attentiveness may be the most important factor in achieving a sense of privacy. The patient needs to feel and to actually be the focus of the nurse's attention and interest.

Noise

Noise often interferes with the transmission of messages, as shown by the following situation. Mrs. Clark is scheduled for a biopsy tomorrow. She has a very soft voice, which is difficult to hear over any noises. She has a roommate who groans intermittently. The nurse has the following options to modify Mrs. Clark's environment: 1. transfer her to a private room if this is economically feasible; 2. transfer the other patient; 3. take Mrs. Clark to a quiet place if she is able; or 4. take advantage of any time the other patient is scheduled to be out of the room. Actions as simple as closing the door or turning off the television can sometimes be helpful. Assessment of the overall situation is essential in selecting the best option. Other hospital noises can be distracting, but the nurse must determine which can be controlled or minimized.

Light

The general level of light in a room is an easily controlled environmental factor that should be managed according to the patient's preference. Dim light may be preferred by some, but it may be a block to communication for others since it tends to obscure the facial expressions of the other person. Nonverbal cues may be an aid to interpretation of the message. If a person is sitting with a light glaring in the eyes, it is difficult for the person to concentrate on the conversation because the light is uncomfortable. Glare tends to blur the words on a printed page. Blinking lights such as those on a monitor tend to divert attention away from the speaker. If the patient is positioned properly, these distractions can be avoided.

Interruptions

Interruptions may ruin a potentially effective communication interaction, as shown in the following situation.

> *Nurse:* You seem to be depressed today.
> *Patient:* Oh, I guess I'll be all right. My husband called and said he is being transferred, and I hate the thought of moving. I'll have to find a new doctor and won't have any friends . . .
> (Technician enters room to draw blood for tests.)
> *Nurse:* (after technician leaves) You mentioned two reasons why you hate to move. What else about the move bothers you?
> *Patient:* Nothing, really. We have moved before. I will be fine. Isn't it about time for lunch? I'm hungry. I do hope they have a good salad. What kind of salads do you like?

It is obvious that the patient will not discuss her concerns about moving at this time. Introducing the topic after lunch or the next day might be more effective. Communication cannot always be scheduled, but it is possible to plan to spend time with a patient when there is the least likelihood of interruptions.

Time of Day

The time of day chosen to initiate communication with a patient can make a difference. Many persons tend to be more responsive during nursing care since the communication seems more casual and not the main focus of the nurse's attention. Patients are often more responsive in the morning than later in the day, but this does not always hold true. Some may prefer talking in the evening after visiting hours, when the tempo of the hospital slows. If a patient has few visitors, communication during visiting hours may be ideal. After lunch is not usually a good time because many people tend to be drowsy after a meal. Each patient must be assessed to determine the optimum time of day in which to initiate meaningful communication.

Effect of Status of Patient on Communication

Background Factors

Age and *developmental level* are variables that must be considered. Communication with a child is approached differently than with an adult. Baby talk must not be used with children, but any explanations must be given in very simple terms. This would also hold true for an adult who happened to have a developmental level of a normal 6-year-old child. It certainly would not necessarily be true for an elderly person, even though the late years are sometimes referred to as a second childhood. Communication with the elderly must be maintained on the same level as with younger adults.

Assessment of an individual's *cultural background* promotes understanding of language usage. While no dialect is considered deficient, some are not considered standard. Communication must be within the framework of the patient's background. The language usage must be accepted, and all communication with the other person must be in understandable language. A person of another culture should not be approached on a childish level, but generally accepted terminology should be used. Unfamiliar phrases used by the other person should be clarified in a nonjudgmental manner.

The *level of education* of patients tends to influence the manner in which the nurse communicates with them. This is reflected more in terminology used than in grammatical structure. If aware that a person has only a fourth-grade education, the effective communicator uses simpler language. For example, instead of, "This medication will relieve your abdominal discomfort," a statement such as, "This pill will make your stomach feel better," would probably be better understood. The nurse must be careful not to talk down to a person who has had limited educational opportunities.

Verbal ability is not always linked to level of education. Some persons with little education may be able to express themselves more eloquently than others with more years of formal education. Verbal ability can be determined only by face-to-face communication. Encouraging communication enables the nurse to assess the verbal ability of the patient and from this knowledge to communicate more effectively with that individual.

Physiological Status

The current physiological status of the patient has an effect on ability to communicate. A very ill patient does not have the energy required to communicate. Responses may be different from those normally elicited, and short answers may be given to end the conversation as soon as possible. Pain and pain medication can cause any message to be blurred. Physical status must be assessed to avoid causing the patient undue exertion and to determine the appropriate time to initiate communication.

Sensory deficits may interfere with transmission of messages. When there is a loss of hearing, messages may be misheard. "The doctor said you can go home," may be heard as, "The doctor said you have no hope." This would undoubtedly have a tremendous impact on the patient. The nurse must first assess hearing status, then validate the message received by assessing the patient's feedback. Related factors might be that the batteries in a hearing aid need replacing or that the family has failed to bring the hearing aid to the hospital. Visual deficits can be a source of difficulty in communication as related to observing nonverbal behaviors and use of any written materials. The deficit may be a physical impairment or the fact that the patient's glasses are not available.

Physiological factors not directly related to health status, such as drowsiness, hunger, or thirst, can act as blocks to communication. These basic needs must be identified and met before the mind is ready to concentrate on communication.

Emotional Factors

All emotions tend to influence the ability to communicate at a given time. When emotionally upset, a person tends to misunderstand messages, to take a slight change in schedule as a sign of rejection, or to become angered when requests are not immediately granted. Anger produces words not normally said. Anxiety tends to let people hear what they want and block out those things they would rather not hear. It can cause a person to misunderstand a message to mean the opposite of what was intended and not as the person would normally interpret it. In discussing an upcoming relatively minor surgery, but one about which the patient feels some anxiety, the nurse's statement, "I think you'll be back in your room by noon," might be interpreted as, *Thinks* I'll be back here by noon—not even sure I'll get back." An effective communicator should strive to understand the meaning behind responses and encourage the patient to verbalize feelings.

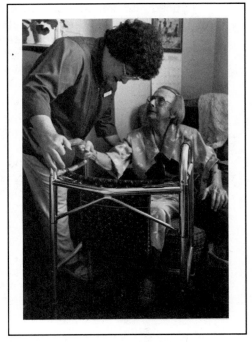

Effect of Behaviors of the Nurse on Communication

Active Listening

The process of active listening was explored in detail in the preceding chapter. It is mentioned again to emphasize the importance of listening in the communication process. Active listening notes the nonverbal as well as the verbal message of the speaker, any discrepancies between the two, and implied feelings apart from the content of the message. Through the process of active listening, the nurse conveys interest, caring, empathy, and other positive aspects of a nurse-patient relationship that contribute to effective, therapeutic communication.

Following Through on Cues

A cue is a signal or a hint; it indicates the nature of something perceived. Failure to pick up on cues is one of the most common weaknesses in communication. Student nurses, as well as many practicing nurses, find it difficult to discuss some concerns of the patient and may ignore cues to these concerns. The following example illustrates this. Mrs. Thurmond has been in the hospital for the past 3 weeks. Two years ago the doctor discovered a malignant tumor in her kidney. At surgery it was discovered that the cancer had spread; the condition is now considered terminal. The nurse is bathing her this morning.

> *Nurse:* You seem to be feeling stronger this morning.
> *Mrs. T.:* Well, in a way.
> *Nurse:* Your face has more color in it.
> *Mrs. T.:* I know that I don't have much longer to live and I want to make all the arrangements that I can before I die.
> *Nurse:* Oh, you may respond well to chemotherapy and have several more years.
> *Mrs. T.:* I don't think so.
> *Nurse:* I believe breakfast trays are here. I'll go get yours.

The nurse ignored these very evident verbal cues, perhaps because talking about death was uncomfortable. Here is an example of following through on a nonverbal cue the same patient may have given.

> *Nurse:* How are you feeling this morning?
> *Mrs. T.:* Fine. (She turns away with a frown on her face.)
> *Nurse:* You seem depressed this morning.
> *Mrs. T.:* I guess I am.
> *Nurse:* Do you want to talk about it?
> *Mrs. T.:* I would like to but no one seems to want to listen when I mention dying.
> *Nurse:* (taking patient's hand) I'll talk with you about whatever you like.

In this example Mrs. Thurmond verbalizes that she is fine, but the nonverbal communication is not congruent. By following through on the cue, the nurse enables Mrs. Thurmond to express her feelings. Death may be a difficult subject for nurses to deal with, but it is one that terminally ill patients may need to discuss. This requires communication expertise and compassion on the part of the nurse.

Not only terminally ill patients, but any patient may make a reference to personal problems, such as family problems, and need a listening ear. Most patients are not trying to find someone to solve problems or give advice; their main concern often is to be able to talk about their problem in an effort to find the answer.

CHECK IT OUT

In a patient assignment assess your behaviors that promoted communication. What did you do to make the environment conducive to effective communication? What specific behaviors indicated that you were listening? Did you pick up and follow through on any cues?

Answer the questions honestly. Try to correct any areas in which you believe you were not effective.

Suspending Judgment

Tolerance is a true virtue. An effective communicator does not judge others but accepts them as they are. Prejudice is a preformed judgment of others; it is always negative, an opinion adverse to something or someone without just grounds or before sufficient knowledge is obtained. Prejudice is not pleasant in any society but has always been a part of human relations.

Prejudice may be thought of as an adult attitude, but it is one that is transmitted to children at an early age by parents and/or significant others. Racial, ethnic, or religious prejudices may be reinforced by peer groups as the child moves into larger circles outside of the family or they may be discarded as the older child makes friends with members of diverse groups.

Persons with prejudices tend to group or classify people, to stereotype them. Stereotyped groups are not restricted to racial, ethnic, and cultural groups. They may be related to socioeconomic status or to occupation. Any general classification used reflects an attitude; no category is without an element of subjectivity. Persons with prejudices look for certain traits in groups and read into behaviors those traits expected, ignoring anything that does not coincide with the stereotyped picture. Preconceived judgments always block interpersonal communication.

Value judgments and prejudice are related in that neither is based on factual evidence. In making value judgments, individuals apply their own standards or value systems to judge another person or situation. Each individual has a different background and a different value system. Value judgments involve the imposition of one person's standards on another, basing opinions on personal experiences rather than considering the other person's experiences and total situation. Making a value judgment of another person is usually obvious to the other person. It creates an attitude toward another that is reflected in all communication, resulting in a negative attitude that can destroy a relationship as well as block communication.

FACILITATIVE TECHNIQUES IN COMMUNICATION

Facilitative techniques are types of responses used to make communication easier, to encourage the other person to verbalize thoughts and feelings, and to achieve effective therapeutic communication. The techniques enable the nurse to help patients feel better about themselves. Effective communication requires some planning, although much of it is spontaneous and will occur during nursing care. The planning is in a nonspecific manner; the nurse assesses the patient to determine the best overall approach. The planning is directed toward the ends to be achieved by the interaction rather than specifics. Any communication interaction must be flexible; the patient's cues must be considered and the general status of the patient taken into account. Facilitative techniques involve nonverbal as well as verbal components. The following paragraphs emphasize some of the major verbal techniques that encourage communication.

Open-Ended Questions/Statements

The nurse seeks to understand the patient's perception of a problem and the ability to cope with it by encouraging discussion. Questions are essential to determine the problems and concerns of the patient. Questioning gives the nurse needed informa- tion and provides an opportunity for the patient to discuss concerns. Questions are not only the most commonly used but also abused technique in nurse-patient interactions. Some questions, especially "why" questions, tend to put the patient on the defensive. This type of question implies that the patient has done something wrong. Open-ended questions—"what," "when," "where," and "how" questions— require more than one or two words for an answer. They cannot be answered by a "yes" or "no." Examples of open-ended questions to obtain information are: "How did you sleep last night?" and "What would you like to talk about today?"

An open-ended statement such as "Tell me what you want to discuss," or "I'd like to hear more about your problem," allows the patient to determine the general direction of the conversation. The nurse may indicate a topic, such as "Tell me about your last hospitalization," or "Tell me what you need to know about your diet." Open- ended statements may be useful in referring back to a topic the patient has mentioned but not elaborated upon, such as "You were telling me a little about . . ." This statement focuses on patient concerns when the conversation has drifted away or when the patient has changed the subject. Open-ended questions and statements, especially general ones, give patients more control over communica- tion, thus helping to maintain a feeling of independence.

Clarifying

To clarify is to make clear, to free of confusion. Clarification of messages is essential for effective communication. This may be simply a matter of asking the other person to repeat what was said, or it may be more involved when confirming the perception of the message. The clarification of messages is a two-way street in which each participant has the opportunity to clear up any misperceptions and avoid misunderstandings. The nurse conveys an attitude of wanting to understand without implying criticism of the manner in which patients express themselves. Techniques useful in clarifying messages include reflecting, paraphrasing, se- quencing, and summarizing.

Reflecting

The use of reflection involves the repetition of all or part of messages. It allows the patient to reevaluate the message and to know that the nurse is trying to under- stand. Reflection is especially useful in helping the patient express feelings because it tends to stimulate elaboration of areas that have been vaguely ex- pressed. For example, Mr. Ingram has been hospitalized for 2 weeks. His wife has been unable to visit often since she works full time and cares for their three preschool children.

> *Mr. I.:* No one cares anything about me.
> *Nurse:* No one cares anything about you?
> *Mr. I.:* Well, if they did they would come to see me.

The nurse has repeated Mr. Ingram's words. It has helped him to express the reason he feels unloved and, hopefully, will open the door to a fuller expression of feelings.

Reflecting may be selective, that is, only parts of the statement may be repeated. Selective reflection pinpoints a specific part of the message.

> *Mr. I.:* I don't know why they're doing all of these tests. I think they are a waste of time and cost a lot of money.
> *Nurse:* You don't know why?
>   Or   A waste of time?
>   Or   Cost a lot of money?

This "selective reflecting" allows the nurse to focus on the part of the statement that seems to be the most pertinent. Reflection stimulates reevaluation on the part of the patient. The first response may help Mr. Ingram to express his understanding of the illness. The second may help him express his attitude toward the doctor and the health care facility. The third response focuses on his financial status and could lead to assistance in securing financial aid if needed. In this example, selective reflection seems more appropriate than a reflection of the entire statement, since three different thoughts are expressed.

Reflection often focuses on feelings and acts like a mirror to help the sender "hear" the message as it is spoken by another person. This allows the sender to clarify or possibly reevaluate the message. Reflection enables the listener to verify the message received and shows a positive regard for the patient by communicating a desire to understand.

Reflection can be a very effective technique if not overused. Too frequent and indiscriminate use of reflection can serve as a block rather than as a facilitator. The patient may get the impression that the nurse is not listening, only mimicking statements in a preoccupied manner.

Paraphrasing

Paraphrasing is a restatement of the message using different words. In the preceding situation, the nurse might have paraphrased a response to Mr. Ingram's statement regarding the tests by saying, "You don't understand the tests?" Paraphrasing is sometimes considered a form of reflection but differs in that the message is rephrased. This response must use simple, precise, and relevant terms by which the interpretation of the patient's message is clarified. For example:

> *Patient:* I tossed and turned all night.
> *Nurse:* You weren't able to sleep last night?

The nurse has interpreted the patient's message as the inability to sleep. This may or may not be correct; the message may have indicated that discomfort tended to rouse the patient from sleep at intervals. The patient's response should indicate the correctness of the nurse's interpretation. Regardless, the patient is made aware of what the nurse is thinking about the message and that someone is listening and trying to understand.

Paraphrasing gives a clear perception of the nurse's interpretation of the patient's message. It is based on empathy as the nurse tries to understand the patient's feelings. It may amplify the meaning of the message or highlight the content. It is a facilitative technique that can be utilized by most nurses without difficulty.

CHECK IT OUT

In talking with a friend, use reflection and paraphrasing no more than two times. Was it effective in promoting communication?
In another conversation with this or another friend, use reflection and/or paraphrasing repeatedly. What was the response after repeated usage?
Facilitators must be used with discretion to be effective.

Sequencing

Sequencing simply means placing events in a time sequence. Patients sometimes relate a series of events out of order, making it difficult to understand or to determine a plan for care. The following illustrates the use of sequencing. Mrs. Jarrod experienced a fall while hospitalized and was relating the incident to the nurse.

> *Mrs. J.:* I had to go to the bathroom so I got up. I told the nurse I had a headache and took a pain pill because she wouldn't give me one. The doctor prescribed them about a month ago and I still had some in my purse. I know when I have a headache and need one even if she said it wasn't time. My headache is better now because I know what I need.
>
> *Nurse:* You asked for something for pain, but the nurse said it was too soon. You took a tablet that you had in your purse then fell when you got up.

The nurse placed the events in a logical time order to gain a clearer perspective of the situation. This clarified the circumstances leading up to the fall. Sequencing is useful in establishing factors precipitating pain. For example, the patient may give a rather rambling account of abdominal pain. By sequencing the related events with, "You pain is severe after meals?" the nurse helps to pinpoint an important factor.

Summarizing

Restating in a summary fashion is another method of clarifying. It may be likened to a chapter summary in a book. It is a statement of the important points in a brief form which unifies the main themes of content or feeling. Summarizing promotes mutual understanding between patient and nurse as the nurse highlights data perceived as significant. The patient may be relating a previous hospital experience.

> *Patient:* I had surgery 2 years ago and swore I'd never go through it again. It hurt to move a single muscle. I was sick to my stomach for days, and I didn't feel like myself again for 6 months. The thought of being cut open again sends shivers down my spine.
>
> *Nurse:* You experienced a lot of pain and discomfort following your last surgery and are apprehensive of another surgery.

The nurse has summarized the patient's account and could open the door for the patient to explore feelings of fear regarding any anticipated surgery. The nurse accepts the patient's feelings in a nonjudgmental manner in an attempt to place the past experiences in proper perspective. It is often helpful for the patient to hear a summary of a conversation because it ties together several ideas and/or feelings to clarify what has been said. It allows the patient to verify or to modify the nurse's perceptions.

Validating

To validate means to confirm and to establish truth or accuracy. Validation, like clarification, helps assure mutual understanding because it involves identifying what one person believes the other person is trying to communicate and asking if that is correct. Validation differs from clarification in that it involves interpretation of nonverbal as well as verbal communication. Note the validation of a verbal message in the following situation.

> *Mr. Fox:* That pill I took just now didn't look like the ones I've been taking.
> *Nurse:* Are you saying that you were given the wrong medication?

Mr. Fox has the opportunity to agree with the nurse's statement or to say that the pill looked different but that he might be wrong.

In other situations the cues may be only nonverbal. Mrs. Bradford has been recently diagnosed as having diabetes and has been discharged. She attended all of the diabetic classes at the hospital and responded well in the group situation. The nurse is helping Mrs. Bradford get her belongings together to go home. She is frowning and her hands are shaking as she picks up the insulin bottle and syringes.

> *Mrs. B.:* Well, I have been practicing this. (The equipment slips from her hand as she reaches for her purse.) Oh dear, clumsy me. I'll be okay when I get home. I have these directions. (Folding and unfolding some papers.)
> *Nurse:* You seem uncertain of being able to care for yourself at home.

Though the cues were not verbal, they were quite obvious. This gives Mrs. Bradford an opening to discuss her concerns about discharge if the nurse's interpretation is correct and to deny her uncertainty if she feels confident about her ability to care for herself.

Validation requires good listening and observation skills. It is essential to hear the words as well as what is between the words, the paralanguage, and the nonverbal indicators. As the nurse is validating the patient's messages during an interchange, the patient may be validating the nurse's responses. Look at a possible situation. Mr. Crow is a 72-year-old man who has been hospitalized for the first time. He is scheduled for a GI series in the morning. The nurse on the evening shift stops in his room.

> *Nurse:* Hi. How is it going this afternoon?
> *Mr. C.:* What does it matter? (He seems upset.)
> *Nurse:* I have some time and thought I'd visit with you.
> *Mr. C.:* (I wonder if she means it.) I'm not going anywhere.
> *Nurse:* (sitting beside bed) Do you mind if I sit down?
> *Mr. C.:* Are you going to take time to sit here and talk to me?
> *Nurse:* Yes, because you seem upset.

This should be the start of an effective, therapeutic interaction. Each person validated the message of the other, verbal and nonverbal. Validation provides mutual understanding between patient and nurse and helps build a positive relationship.

Acknowledging Feelings

Many people try to hide their feelings to keep others from knowing when something causes anxiety or from realizing when they are depressed, lonely, or afraid. Revealing feelings may be considered a sign of weakness by some people. However, everyone experiences numerous emotions in varying degrees. To be unable to share feelings tends to magnify negative feelings and to minimize positive ones. Whether feelings are expressed, implied, or sensed by the nurse, they should be acknowledged. The acknowledgement is an expression of empathy and creates an opening for further exploration. Consider the following interactions.

> *Patient:* I am really concerned about the surgery for fear that it may be cancer.
> *Nurse:* I'm quite certain I would be very worried.

The feeling has been openly expressed and acknowledged by the nurse.

> *Patient:* I'll be glad when this surgery is over.
> *Nurse:* I'm sure I would be quite anxious about it.

The anxiety is acknowledged by the nurse even though it is not openly expressed but implied.

> *Patient:* (Staring out of window, frowning with hands clasped tightly together. Surgery is scheduled for tomorrow.)
> *Nurse:* You seem to be worried. I know you must be anxious about your surgery tomorrow.

The feeling has not been expressed or implied, but the nurse assesses the nonverbal cues. In each of these situations the nurse has verbally acknowledged a perception of the feelings of the patient and has followed through on the verbal, implied, and nonverbal cues. This acknowledgement of the patient's feelings encourages further exploration, a mark of effective communication.

Reassuring

Everyone wants and needs reassurance. Children want to be reassured that parents will not leave them; students need reassurance of passing grades in courses; wives and husbands want periodic reassurance that their spouse still loves them; and the elderly want to be reassured that someone will look after them. Patients have definite needs for reassurance, and giving them reassurance is an important aspect of nursing care.

But what are the areas in which the nurse can give patients reassurance? Patients can be reassured that someone is there to care for them, that someone is listening and understands their problem, that they are seen as individuals, or that there is hope for their recovery even though it may be a lengthy process in some instances. However, to reassure terminal cancer patients that they will be able to return home and resume former activities is an insult to their intelligence. By reassuring patients in a straightforward, honest way the nurse can confirm their self-worth and create a sense of hope.

The nurse can reassure the patient verbally that, for example, the ability to function independently will be regained.

> *Mrs. Long:* It's been 3 weeks since I had that surgery on my knee and I still can't walk alone. I can't do my housework if I have to keep using this walker.
>
> *Nurse:* I know it must seem like a long time to you, Mrs. Long, but you have made a lot of progress. Within another few weeks you should be able to walk with only a cane and gradually be able to walk without an aid.

The nurse can reassure patients nonverbally by smiling, by maintaining active listening postures, by answering call lights promptly, by being receptive to what patients have to say, and by using touch. Whatever approach is used to reassure the patient, it should clearly communicate the intended message.

Silence

The communication techniques discussed have involved a verbal element. Verbal skills are important, but silence can also be a very effective technique. People who find silence uncomfortable and fill any gap with conversation may find it difficult to utilize silence. A break in verbal communication gives both participants time to reflect on what has been said, time to process the information. It allows the patient time to select the right words to express thoughts or feeings, and it conveys that the nurse is interested enough to wait for an answer. Silence can also give the nurse time to regroup and determine the best approach in the particular situation. But silence can be overused the same as any of the communication techniques. It can be a result of tuning out the other person, not knowing what to say, or not having anything to say.

Silence may create anxiety in patients who are not comfortable with it. Any cue indicating discomfort during a silence, such as facial muscles tensing, should be noted by the nurse and an appropriate response made, such as, "What were you about to say?" The lapse in verbal communication should never be used by the nurse to change the subject. Silences do not have to be long to be effective. A 10- to 15-second interval can be quite effective. It can be a time to share another's company and a thoughtful period of reflection, giving a warm feeling to both parties.

COMMUNICATION BLOCKS

Ideally, channels of communication are never blocked but remain open for messages to flow without restrictions. Unfortunately, this is not always true. Just as a water drain can become clogged or an artery in the body blocked, so channels of communication may be blocked. In nurse-patient interactions the nurse may fail to apply effective communication techniques, the patient may consciously or unconsciously block communication, or an outside factor may break the flow of communication. Awareness of potential blocks enhances the nurse's ability to communicate effectively.

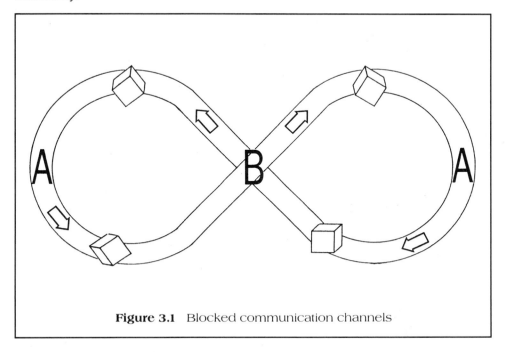

Figure 3.1 Blocked communication channels

Nurses may block communication without realizing it. Responses that tend to block communication are those that indicate a lack of interest in what is being said, that tend to lower self-esteem, or that seem to close the topic being discussed. While the use of one block will not necessarily destroy the effectiveness of a communication interaction, it will make it more difficult to achieve the intended result.

Closed-Ended Questions

Questions that can be answered with a "yes" or "no" as well as those requiring only one- or two-word responses are considered closed-ended. Sometimes this type of question will be answered at length by the other participant, even though the question did not act as a facilitator. Closed-ended questions are easily reworded to be open-ended.

Closed: Are you feeling better this morning?
Open: How are you feeling this morning?
Closed: Do you think the medication will help you?
Open: What is your opinion of the medication?

Closed-ended questions may be considered a potential, not definite, block since they do not always interrupt the flow of communication.

CHECK IT OUT

Reword the following closed-ended questions to make them open-ended.
Are you making progress with your walker?
When did you move to this city?
Didn't you go to therapy yesterday?
How many children do you have?
Did you take your medicine this morning?

Clichés

Clichés are trite, hackneyed phrases, unoriginal and overused. They appear in everyday conversations in such forms as, "You're the greatest," or "Tomorrow will be better." They have become almost meaningless from overuse as a substitute for anything better to say. Clichés have a negative effect because they are interpreted by the patient as an impersonal expression devoid of any concern on the part of the nurse. The following example illustrates this. Mr. Patman is scheduled for surgery tomorrow.

> *Mr. P.:* The thought of being cut open tomorrow really has me nervous.
> *Nurse:* Just keep your chin up.

Mr. Patman's statement indicates a need to express his feelings and talk about the surgery. He may feel that any further attempt to discuss the surgery would be interpreted as a sign of weakness. This cliché definitely ended the communication.

False or Inappropriate Reassurance

Reassurance that takes into consideration probable outcomes was a communication facilitator noted previously. However, false or inappropriate reassurance does not take the probable outcome into consideration but paints a rosy picture regardless of the facts. It may be an attempt to cheer up the patient, but it does not accomplish this purpose.

> *Nurse:* How are you today?
> *Mr. Jones:* Not any better. Just don't know if I ever will be able to go back to work.
> *Nurse:* Sure. You will be back on the job in no time.

The nurse is disregarding Mr. Jones' feelings of the moment. It may be true that the possibility of Mr. Jones' eventual recovery from the illness is good, but this response blocks any discussion of the illness. Mr. Jones may have a need to express anxieties and fears but thinks that the nurse does not want to try to understand his feelings. False reassurance is especially traumatic to the terminally ill patient, for example:

> *Mrs. Cass:* The doctor told me that I probably won't be able to go home again.

> *Nurse:* You are doing so much better that you'll be back home and on your feet real soon.

Mrs. Cass had been diagnosed as having cancer 3 years ago. The cancer has now metastasized to numerous organs. She needs someone with whom to talk about her fears and anxieties, but the opportunity has not been provided by this nurse. This may raise a question as to whether the nurse or the patient receives the most benefit from false reassurance.

Judgmental Responses

Judgmental responses are similar to value judgments in that both involve opinions based on personal value systems. Judgmental responses, however, are opinions expressed regarding a specific situation or a response to a statement. These expressed opinions imply right or wrong in regard to the statement or aspect of a situation. They are not an overall judgment of the individual. The judgmental response tends to block communication because it says, in effect, "That's how it is," which leaves no room for further discussion.

Stating one's own opinion (agree/disagree; approve/disapprove)

The statement of an opinion tends to indicate that one viewpoint is right and the other wrong. The opinion of one person may agree with that of the other person or approve of that person's actions, or it may be negative and disapprove of proposed actions or disagree with a statement. By using these responses, the nurse is in effect saying that the patient does or does not measure up to expectations. The patient may be uncertain about a personal decision and seeking an answer. For example, Mrs. Coy has been hospitalized as the result of a beating from her husband.

> *Mrs. C.:* I think I will see a laywer about a divorce as soon as I get out of here.
> *Nurse:* You are doing the right thing. A woman should not live with a man who mistreats her.

While Mrs. Coy is in the hospital, her husband seeks help and is going to counseling sessions regularly. She feels that he has made tremendous progress and that his attitude toward her has changed. She would like to talk to the nurse about this but is hesitant because she fears the nurse will disapprove of the possibility of her going back to her husband.

Disapproving places the patient in a position similar to that of approving or agreeing. It prevents the patient from sharing feelings that might bring a reprimand. For example, Mrs. Klaus has two teenagers at home who have had a minimum of supervision since she has been in the hospital.

> *Mrs. K.:* I just hope my children are eating right while I'm in here.
> *Nurse:* You shouldn't worry about them. They can take care of themselves. You should just think about getting well.

Should and should not have no place in effective communication. With this expression of disapproval by the nurse, Mrs. Klaus is reluctant to share any other feelings. Feelings are not correct or incorrect, good or bad; they need no label. They are something that may be shared with another person, but only if the other person has proven capable of accepting the knowledge without being judgmental.

Giving Advice

Advising deals with individual choice rather than an expert opinion. In nurse-patient communication advising tends to place the patient in a parent/child position. The patient may see the nurse as "the professional" and attempt to follow the advice. Or the advice given by the nurse may not be the same as that from another source, which tends to cause the patient additional concern. For example, Mr. Adkins is to be discharged from the hospital tomorrow following a total hip replacement.

> *Mr. A:* I'm not sure my wife will be able to take care of me at home.
> *Nurse:* I think you should go to a nursing home for awhile and not take any chances.

Mrs. Adkins has made arrangements for some help at home and feels confident of being able to care for her husband. Although Mr. Adkins needs some additional information regarding care at home, he is reluctant to ask this nurse since he is not following the advice given. A much better approach by the nurse would have been to explore Mr. Adkins' options for care following discharge. This would leave the door open for current and future interactions.

Belittling

Belittling tends to lower another person's self-esteem. It is a cruel response in any communication interaction and has no place in effective nurse-patient relationships. It is minimizing the seriousness of a problem and is disparaging to the individual.

> *Patient:* I have never been this sick before.
> *Nurse:* Lots of patients here are much sicker than you are.

This statement may have been an attempt on the part of the nurse to convince the patient that chances for recovery were good, but it would probably be interpreted by the patient to mean that the nurse did not believe that this illness was very serious. It would definitely preclude further sharing of feelings by the patient. Belittling is a type of blocker that does irreparable damage to the patient as well as to the communication process.

Stereotyping the Individual

Stereotyping may be considered a type of value judgment because a judgment has been made that places the individual in a particular category. Stereotyping stems from prejudice; it ignores individual differences and automatically makes the assumption that the person possesses the characteristics of the stereotype. The following situation illustrates this.

> *Mrs. Cass:* I hope my husband is still interested in going to bed with me after this mastectomy.
> *Nurse:* A 68-year-old woman doesn't need to be concerned with sex appeal.

The nurse has neatly categorized Mrs. Cass according to her age and erroneously assumed that older adults are not interested in sex. Stereotypes are similar to prejudice but do not always carry the negative connotations of prejudice. Patients may be stereotyped as good or difficult, age groups may be given specific characteristics, and occupations may be considered worthwhile or demeaning. Regardless of whether the stereotype carries a positive or negative connotation, the individual differences are not taken into account.

Defending

Defending is a type of communication block that is made as a response to a feeling of being threatened. The nurse may feel threatened in a direct or indirect manner. Defending may be a response intended as a defense of another nurse, a doctor, or the hospital. Defensive responses may lead to an argument between a nurse and patient that will not benefit anyone and may lead to disciplinary action against the nurse. The effective communicator avoids this type of response. Even through there is no hint of an argument, a defensive response causes the patient to be reluctant to express feelings. For example, Mrs. Lang had surgery 2 days ago. She is doing well but had difficulty sleeping last night. She had requested an additional sleeping medication but the nurse told her it could not be repeated.

> *Mrs. L.:* That nurse last night just didn't care how I felt. She wouldn't give me any medicine when I asked for it.
> *Nurse:* The nurses on this staff are excellent and take very good care of you.

Mrs. Lang was quite upset and further embellished the story when the doctor visited that morning.

This misunderstanding could easily have been avoided. How much better it would have been if the communication had evolved more in the following manner:

> *Mrs. L.:* That nurse last night just didn't care how I felt. She wouldn't give me any medicine when I asked for it.
> *Nurse:* What medicine did you ask her about?
> *Mrs. L.:* That pill to make me sleep.
> *Nurse:* Tell me what you had taken before that.
> *Mrs. L.:* I had a pain pill and a sleeping tablet at bedtime but woke up at 4 o'clock and couldn't go back to sleep. I wasn't really hurting.
> *Nurse:* The doctor does not want sleeping tablets repeated. If you had taken another one at 4 o'clock this morning, you would probably have slept all day.
> *Mrs. L.:* That's a point. But the night gets so long when I can't sleep.

With this as a beginning the interaction could progress to the point of a fuller expression of feelings by the patient and a greater understanding by the nurse.

Challenging

An almost certain way to block communication is to challenge the other participant. Challenging demands an explanation. It forces the other person to prove a point of view. In the process of challenging it is rare for participants to change their minds; in fact their point of view may even be strengthened. Challenging may be a response to a patient's complaint. Challenging, which is questioning the validity of the patient's statement, goes one step further than defending. For example,

> *Patient:* I don't seem to be getting any better. I wonder if the doctor has
> seen many cases like mine before.
> *Nurse:* Well, maybe you should ask the doctor about that. I suppose you
> know what treatment is needed.

This response indicates that the nurse is on the opposing side; it negates any idea of the nurse as patient advocate.

Any patient complaints should be considered seriously even though the nurse does not agree with the basis of the grievance. Some complaints may not be valid, but the well-being of the patient must be the first consideration. For example, Miss Bonner is an 18-year-old only child from an affluent family who is accustomed to immediate gratification of any request. The previous evening she had asked for a soft drink that was not available on the unit. It was about 20 minutes before one of the staff could go to another floor to obtain the drink from a machine. As the nurse was taking care of her the following morning, Miss Bonner complained about the incident.

> *Miss B.:* It just takes forever to get anything around here. It was
> practically bedtime before I could get a simple little soft drink that I
> had asked for much earlier.
> *Nurse:* What makes you think you are the only patient here?

The patient's immediate reaction would probably be one of anger. The consequences of this challenging response will not be beneficial to anyone. A calm inquiry into the specifics of the complaint and a discussion of ways in which a similar situation could be avoided would benefit both participants. Challenging responses always act as a block and should be avoided.

Changing the Subject

A change of subject may indicate that there is nothing further to say on the subject or that there is a lack of interest in the present discussion. It is a type of defensive reaction when the person is not comfortable with the topic. Introducing another topic after one has been explored is not the same as changing the subject abruptly. The following is an example of this type of block.

> *Patient:* I have been in this bed so long that I may not be able to walk
> when they let me up.
> *Nurse:* Sure, you will. Is your daughter coming to see you this evening?

The patient's concern was ignored and an unrelated topic introduced, which conveys a lack of interest in the patient. The nurse may have changed the subject because of feeling unprepared to discuss the concerns. But extensive knowledge of expected outcome or specifics of care is not necessary for discussion. If the patient has questions that the nurse is unable to answer, finding the answer from another source is not difficult. The average patient does not expect the nurse to have all the answers but does expect the nurse to communicate.

CHECK IT OUT

In general conversations with friends, note and identify any blocks used by the other person. How did you respond to the block? Deliberately use one or more blocks. How did the other person respond? Remember that some blocks will be ignored and the interaction will continue. Be prepared to discuss in class.

This discussion on communication blocks may tend to inhibit the desire to communicate with patients. The communication process is sensitive but not threatening. The nurse need not fear making a mistake because most mistakes in communication can be corrected. If the nurse has inadvertently blocked an interaction, it is always possible to say, "I'm sorry. I did not mean that the way it may have sounded." This approach will usually be accepted since everyone makes a mistake occasionally.

Communication skills are sharpened with practice. Through application of facilitators and recognition of blocks and potential blocks to communication, the ability to be an effective communicator is strengthened. Evaluating communication interactions to assess positive and negative responses, then making an effort to avoid the blocks and incorporate the facilitative responses in the future promotes communication ability.

The Patient May Block Communication

Patients as well as nurses may block communication. They may introduce an unrelated topic to consciously block a subject they do not wish to discuss. Patients may minimize feedback by giving as brief a response as possible to any attempts at communication. This often indicates that they do not wish to talk about anything at this time. Their nonverbal behavior may indicate that communication is not desired at this time. It may consist of a deliberate turning away from the nurse, a frown on the face when a response is expected, or a pretense of reading or watching television. These nonverbal cues speak loudly and should be respected just as words would be.

Regardless of the method used by the patient, the nurse must accept the fact that the patient does not wish to talk at this time and respect this wish. There are occasions when everyone prefers to be alone, to think through personal problems, or to contemplate future plans. The patient needs to know that the nurse is available and ready to listen whenever the patient is ready to talk. Later approaches to communication with the use of facilitative techniques will often reveal the reason for the earlier communication being blocked.

NEUTRAL COMMUNICATION

Neutral communication is an integral part of communication, even though the responses are neither facilitative nor blocking. Humor is included because it can facilitate or block communication: the discussion will emphasize its use as a facilitator. Information giving and social conversations are the parts of nurse-patient communication that are classed as neutral.

Humor

Laughter is often said to be a great medicine. Humor does have a place in the health care setting. However, it should be spontaneous, such as a witty remark, rather than memorized jokes. It is one way to reach out to patients, to help them through their loneliness and fears, and to make them feel better for awhile. Laughter can bring withdrawn patients out of themselves and can bridge a communication gap. Laughter can produce physiological changes such as stimulation of circulation and respiration and can provide the emotional distance needed to deal with stressful situations.

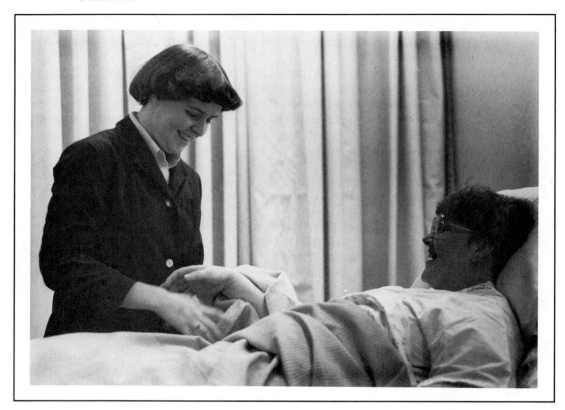

In general the nurse should be receptive and respond to the patient's sense of humor. Jokes may be one of the best weapons against anxiety. However, there may be times when the patient's brand of humor is inappropriate. For instance, sexually suggestive remarks that are passed off as a joke must be rejected.

To be effective, humor must be timely. If the patient needs quiet, needs to be alone, or needs information, humor may be the wrong approach. Humor should not be overused, but a cheerful manner does reassure an anxious patient since it indicates that the situation is under control. Humor should be an adjunct to compassionate care and regard for human dignity. This negates any hint of sarcasm. Humor increases a person's self-esteem; sarcasm and ridicule destroy it.

Humor can also act as a block to communication. A joke at the wrong time or to the wrong person can offend that person. Patients may think their illness is being taken lightly. They may believe that the nurse is laughing at them and not with them. Above all, humor must convey an attitude of caring. If humor does not come naturally, nurses can smile until they develop its use. Humor is a very effective tool that requires some thought and effort in application.

Giving Information

An integral part of the nurse's role as communicator is giving information. This is one of the primary reasons patients list for communicating with nurses. Although not a facilitative technique or a part of therapeutic communication, the nurse acts as an information giver from the time the patient enters the hospital until discharged. The role of the nurse as teacher is that of giving information.

Social Conversation

Socialization is another reason patients frequently list as a reason for communicating with nurses. Social conversation refers to everyday communication with friends and acquaintances, talking about the weather, fashions, what children are doing in school, and who is dating whom. It is a part of relationships with others that is pleasant and interesting. This type of communication is important for getting acquainted with patients and can be very pleasant for both patient and nurse but cannot be considered part of therapeutic communication. It can lead to further communication when the nurse follows through on any cues given by the patient.

INAPPROPRIATE COMMUNICATION

Communication with patients may be inappropriate in the general level of response, in the language used in the interaction, or in the topic itself. Facts may be used inappropriately. If a patient expresses a concern and the nurse responds with facts, the patient will be reluctant to share feelings.

Patient: I hate this tube in my nose. It bothers me and makes me feel like a wimp.

Nurse: The tube goes down to your stomach to minimize gas accumulation and prevent undue stress on your suture line.

The patient's remark was on a feeling level; the nurse responded with facts. While the facts were accurate, the response was inappropriate. The nurse's response would probably block any further expression of concerns by the patient since it did not indicate that the nurse wanted to listen. The language used by the nurse could serve as an additional block if the patient is unfamiliar with medical terminology. A more helpful response by the nurse might have been, "I'm sure it must be most uncomfortable. Tell me how it makes you feel otherwise." This acknowledges the physical discomfort and opens the door for continued expression of feelings.

Questions about intimate details of a patient's personal life are inappropriate unless the answers would be directly related to the current health problem or information that would be used in planning care. The patient may want to share some details; however, this should be the patient's decision with the nurse allowing a free expression of feelings without encouraging details. Anything that the patient might construe as prying would tend to undermine trust in the nurse as well as block communication.

Communication concerning intimate details of the personal life of the nurse is never appropriate in nurse-patient communication. The activities of hospital personnel, except as related to the patient, should not be a topic for discussion. The illness or any other concern of another patient is discussed only with health personnel involved in the patient's care. Communication in these areas removes nurse-patient communication from the realm of professionalism and should be avoided.

IN A CAPSULE

The nurse can create an atmosphere conducive to communication by attention to environmental details such as *general setting, noise, light, interruptions,* and *time of day.* The nurse's general level of communication should be adjusted to the patient's *age and developmental level, cultural background, level of education,* and *verbal ability.* The nurse must consider the patient's *physiological status* and *emotional factors* in initiating communication. The nurse can promote communication by *active listening, following through on cues,* and *suspending judgment.* The elimination of *prejudice,* which leads to stereotyping, must be eliminated for communication to be effective.

Facilitative communication techniques are types of responses that encourage the other person to participate actively in the process of communication. *Open-ended questions and statements* allow the other person to determine the direction of the com

munication. There are several methods of *clarifying* or making clear the content of a message. *Reflecting* is the repetition of all or part of a message. *Paraphrasing* repeats the message in different words. Placing events in a consecutive time frame is termed *sequencing.* In *summarizing,* the information is condensed to make the message clearer. An important communication technique is *validating* or confirming the listener's perception of the message, whether verbal, implied, or nonverbal.

Acknowledging feelings tends to give a sense of sharing and encourages communication. *Reassurance* is a useful technique, but care must be taken to avoid giving false or inappropriate reassurance. A potent technique often overlooked is the use of *silence,* which gives both participants a short time to think.

Closed-ended questions can be answered briefly and do not encourage communication. The use of *clichés* conveys an impersonal attitude in giving a standard answer. *False or inappropriate reassurance* is not based on fact and tends to block further communication. *Judgmental responses* express opinions of situations based on personal value systems. *Stating an opinion* indicates a right and a wrong side, precluding further discussion. *Giving advice* tends to place the other participant in a parent-child position. *Belittling* minimizes situations and lowers the other person's self-esteem. People are placed in categories by *stereotyping*, which ignores all individual differences. A feeling of being threatened may provoke *defending*, which in turn puts the other person on the defensive. A communication block that demands an explanation is *challenging*, which questions the validity of a statement or action. *Changing the subject* is a mechanism frequently used to avoid discussing a topic at that time. *Patients'* wishes should be respected when they *block communication.*

Neutral communication such as giving information and social conversation is an integral part of communication, even though the responses neither facilitate nor block communication. Appropriately used, *humor* can help to establish rapport, but it can also act as a block. *Commnication may be inappropriate* in the level of response, the language used, or the topic introduced.

DO YOU REMEMBER

- patient assessments the nurse should make before initiating communication?
- the impact of the patient's physiological status on communication?
- what is meant by following through on cues?
- the facilitative communication techniques discussed?
- the advantage of open-ended questions and statements?
- the importance of validating your perception of verbal and nonverbal communication?
- how acknowledging feelings and reassurance promote communication?
- the purpose of silence in communication?
- what is meant by a closed-ended question?
- the difference in reassurance and false or inappropriate reassurance?
- the distinction between value judgments and judgmental responses?
- types of communication that are considered neutral?
- what is considered inappropriate communication?

CAN YOU DESCRIBE

- possible modifications in the environment that would promote communication?
- the manner in which emotions affect communication?
- the relationship of prejudice to communication?
- four methods of clarifying a communication message?
- the effect of value judgments on communication?

- how clinchés block communication?
- the four judgmental responses discussed?
- how defending and challenging differ?
- the best approach by the nurse in response to patient blocks to communication?
- the use of humor in communication?

ACTION, PLEASE

1. Change these blockers to facilitators.

   a. Patient: It's taking me so long to get over this surgery.
      Nurse: Well, Rome wasn't built in a day.

      _____

      _____

   b. Patient: I wonder if I should see another doctor.
      Nurse: I think you should see a specialist right away.

      _____

      _____

   c. Patient: It hurts so bad I can't move.
      Nurse: You're being a sissy now.

      _____

      _____

   d. Patient: That last pill I took was blue instead of red.
      Nurse: Our nurses certainly wouldn't give you the wrong medication.

      _____

      _____

2. Watch a short television program with a lot of dialogue. (Soaps are excellent for this.) Note the following:

   a. Program _____

   b. Facilitative techniques used and effectiveness

      _____

      _____

      _____

   c. Blocks noted and response

      _____

      _____

      _____

d. Were any potential blocks ignored? Clarify.

_____

_____

_____

3. *A Communication Situation* Mr. Monroe, a 74-year-old man who has been a widower for less than a year, was admitted to a semiprivate room 2 days ago. Tests revealed an abdominal tumor, and surgery is scheduled for tomorrow. Mr. Monroe has never been hospitalized before and is reluctant to talk to anyone.

a. What environmental arrangements would you make to facilitate communication?

_____

_____

_____

b. How would you initiate communication?

_____

_____

c. What would be your response to, "I don't know how I'll get through this without my wife."?

_____

_____

d. When Mr. Monroe says, "This operation should be real simple," but stammers in getting the words out and is gripping the arms of the chair, how would you validate your perception of the message?

_____

_____

_____

4

Application of Communication Techniques in Nurse-Patient Interactions

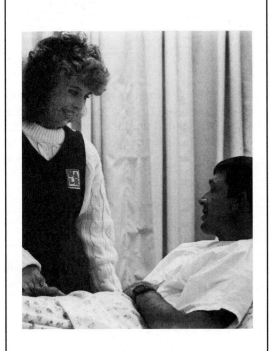

To enjoy life in this world, one must always deal with people, never with things. ***Galiani***

OBJECTIVES

Upon completion of this chapter, the student will be able to:

- differentiate affective and cognitive levels of communication.
- contrast formal and informal communication.
- identify effective uses of social communication.
- discuss applications of goal-directed communication.
- identify essential elements of a goal.
- note parameters and applications of interviews in nurse-patient interactions.
- contrast communication techniques that are most effective with children in different age groups.
- note effective approaches in communicating with the elderly.

- discuss special considerations in communicating with patients who are visually impaired, hearing impaired, terminally ill, dysphasic, speaking a foreign language, or unable to read.
- record a nurse-patient communication interaction and include an evaluation of the technique used.

GLOSSARY OF TERMS*

Affective   Relating to feelings or emotions.

Aphasia   Absence or impairment of the power to communicate as a result of dysfunction of brain centers.

Cognitive   Relating to or based on factual knowledge.

Dysarthria   Difficult and defective speech caused by impairment of tongue or other muscles essential to speech.

Dysphasia   Impairment of speech resulting from brain damage.

Functionally illiterate   Inability to read with sufficient comprehension to function effectively in a complex society.

Goal   The end toward which effort is directed.

Interview   A formal or informal goal-directed interaction conducted primarily at the cognitive level for the purpose of obtaining specific items of information.

Verbatim   Word for word; following the exact words.

*Definitions applicable to content.

The term "nurse-patient communication" has been used frequently in previous chapters. It must be emphasized that nurses communicate with the family as well as with the patient. In some instances the interchanges are almost entirely with the family if the patient's ability to communicate is limited. The approaches and techniques discussed are equally applicable whether communicating with patients or their significant others. This chapter considers some general approaches to communication as well as communicating with patients in special situations. Suggestions for the recording of nurse-patient communication interactions in the clinical setting are included. While this recording may be a time-consuming and seemingly laborious task for students, it is helpful in taking a close look at communication techniques in order to become a more effective communicator.

LEVELS OF COMMUNICATION

Affective Level

The affective level in communication is the feeling or emotional component in an interaction. It deals with feelings about objects, symbols, aspects of our world, or relationships with others. It is the expression of likes or dislikes of people, objects, or situations. It is always influenced by emotions rather than by reasoning. With patients, it often concerns the response to the hospital, the health service personnel, or the particular condition. This reaction may be one of anger, fear, or uncertainty. The patient may express happiness, relief, or sadness at the outcome of tests. The affective component in the behavior of the nurse involves sensitivity to the feelings of the patient.

Cognitive Level

The cognitive level in communication is based on factual knowledge and reasoning. It is the thinking approach without consideration of emotional aspects. Responses may be based on something concrete or abstract, but emotions are not involved. Beliefs, for example, are part of the cognitive domain because they are derived from the thinking process rather than being the result of emotions. Communication is on a cognitive level when a nurse obtains information from the patient for subsequent analysis of data. From the viewpoint of the patient, the seeking and receiving of information is at the cognitive level. The nurse may block communication by responding at the cognitive level when the patient has initiated communication at the affective level, as noted in the discussion on inappropriate communication in the preceding chapter.

TYPES OF COMMUNICATION

Formal Communication

Formal communication is a structured type of communication. Specific items of data are outlined and a sequence followed. This type of communication is frequently scheduled at an appointed time. Notes may be made during the interaction. There are advantages and disadvantages in formal communication. The greatest amount of information can be obtained in the least amount of time, but the personal aspect is lost. Formal communication is useful in the clinical setting to obtain admission information, health histories, and nursing histories. This may be an effective approach in patient teaching when the time factor precludes a less structured approach.

Informal Communication

Informal communication is an unstructured type of communication. There may be a goal and the general area of data to be obtained may be outlined, but specific items are not planned. There is no definite time or place for the interaction, and data are not recorded at the time. The sequence is random rather than patterned. The same information can be obtained through an informal approach as through a formal one, but the length of time required to obtain the information is longer in an informal approach. Informal communication comprises the majority of nurse-patient interactions. It is the approach generally used in obtaining information for nursing assessments and planning of care. Recordings of nurse-patient interactions are based on informal communication. Interactions at the affective level are always informal since it is impossible to anticipate another person's reactions in order to plan the interaction. An informal approach is preferred in orientation of the patient to the hospital setting, even though specific areas of information are included in the orientation.

Social Communication

Social conversation is always an informal type of communication. The time is random, there is no semblance of a pattern, and the environment poses no special problem. It is a definite part of nurse-patient interactions and can fill lonely moments for patients, especially the elderly. The only drawback to this would be if the nurse never progressed beyond socialization in interacting with patients.

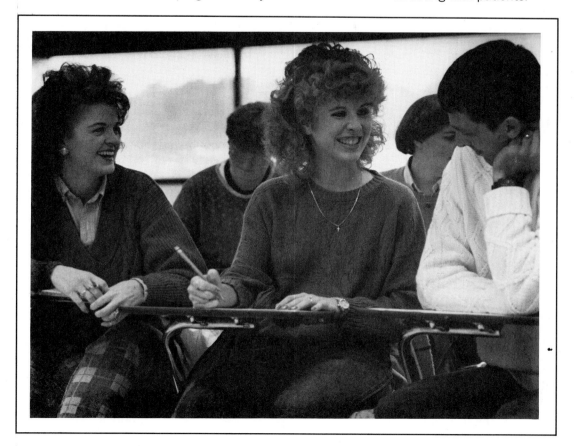

Hospitals may be considered unfriendly and cold places in which nurses seldom socialize. Some persons believe that a successful nurse-patient relationship is a friendly one, while others say that socialization is not advisable in a helping relationship. A successful relationship between nurse and patient differs from the usual definition of friendship. Although it may be a warm and friendly relationship, it is a professional relationship with the purpose of helping rather than an experience designed for mutual enjoyment. Patients may interpret social communication as an expression of nurses caring enough to spend time with them other than that spent in performing nursing procedures. A friendly relationship can be established where there are periods of social conversation without undermining the professional relationship.

Goal-Directed Communication

In this type of communication, there is a definite purpose for the interaction. It is directed toward a specific goal. Planning is often necessary if the goal is to be reached. Goal-directed communication may be formal or informal. It may be at the cognitive or affective level. Formal communication is always goal directed because it is a structured type of communication with a patterned sequence. At the cognitive level, the nurse's goal may be to assess the current status of the patient in order to effectively plan care. Patient teaching is always goal directed. Therapeutic communication is at the affective level, often with a goal relating to the expression of feelings. The course of a therapeutic communication interchange is not patterned but progresses according to patient responses. Nurse-patient communication is frequently goal directed, but only a small portion is formal.

GOALS IN COMMUNICATION

People communicate for a purpose. There may not be a definite goal, but there is always a purpose, even if it is simply to dispel loneliness or to pass the time of day. A goal shows the direction in which we want to be heading. A goal is essential for a person to have a general idea of what is to be accomplished. From a personal viewpoint, goals lead to accomplishment of ambitions, to realization of dreams, to meeting academic requirements, and to full acceptance of professional responsibilities.

To be acceptable, goals must be compatible with values. Values are what one has learned to hold dear, to desire, or to be important in life. Individuals choosing health-related professions tend to place high values on the attainment and maintenance of health. Values, other than basic moral values, are related to understanding. A person does not value matters that are basically unknown or not understood. Conflicts arise if the goals are not compatible with values. The nurse cannot expect the patient to work toward a goal when the importance of attaining it is not understood by the patient.

Short- and Long-Term Goals

Goals may be compared to road maps. The destination can be pinpointed on a map, but the route must be planned to reach the destination. The ultimate destination is the long-term goal and the towns through which one must pass may be likened to short-term goals. Short-term goals should relate to immediate needs and must be accomplishable in a short period of time. Communication situations in which related interactions occur over a period of time may have one long-term goal with several short-term goals for each session. For example, a patient who has been recently diagnosed with cancer refuses to talk about it. A short-term goal might be that the patient will acknowledge the diagnosis. A long-term goal might be that the patient will verbalize feelings regarding the diagnosis. The latter could not be accomplished in a short time.

Essentials of a Goal

If goals are to be effective, they must be mutually acceptable, realistic, measurable, patient centered, within a specific time frame, and written. Many goals in therapeutic communication will be directed toward the affective level, with an emphasis on expression of feelings.

ESSENTIALS OF A GOAL

MUTUALLY ACCEPTABLE
REALISTIC
MEASURABLE
PATIENT CENTERED
TIME FRAME
WRITTEN

Table 4.1 Essentials of a goal

Goals must be *mutually acceptable* to be effective. The patient should have a part in setting the goal, or the nurse must formulate a goal that is acceptable to the patient. For example, the nurse picks up on a cue that indicates that the patient is concerned about upcoming surgery. The nurse sets a goal stating, "The patient will verbalize feelings about the scheduled surgery." The patient did not participate in formulation of the goal, but verbalization indicates acceptance.

The goal must be *realistic*, one that the patient can accomplish. In communication the application of therapeutic techniques may be the key factor in enabling the patient to express feelings if this is the area noted in the goal.

An effective goal must be *measurable*. It must be stated in behavioral terms that can be objectively evaluated.

Goals in any nurse-patient interaction should be *patient centered*. The nurse has goals to be accomplished in regard to the patient, but patient goals should clearly indicate that they are things to be actively accomplished by the patient. For example, consider the following goal statements.

1. Encourage patient to verbalize concerns regarding surgery.
2. Today the patient will verbalize any concerns regarding the surgery scheduled for tomorrow.

They are in essence the same, but the first one is obviously a nursing goal, while the second one emphasizes what the patient is to do. The simplest method of ascertaining that goals are patient centered is to think or state at the beginning of each goal, "the patient will . . ."

An effective goal specifies a *time frame* in which the goal should be met. If no time is specified, it cannot be said that a goal was not met—it may be met the following day.

In many areas such as patient teaching, it is best if goals are *written* to serve as a guideline and provide a basis to evaluate progress. Most communication goals are not written but mentally formulated prior to an interaction as the nurse follows through on cues. At other times the nurse may have one goal in mind when initiating an interaction but will change it during the course of the communication in response to the patient's message.

Goals have been discussed in relation to nurse-patient communication, since this is the emphasis in this unit. But goals are not only reserved for nurse-patient communication. Goals are important in the nursing process and in patient teaching. The principles of goal setting discussed are applicable in other situations as well.

CHECK IT OUT

Read the goals listed below: note those that are stated correctly. Specify any "essential" that is missing and make necessary corrections in the others. The goals may be correct even though "the patient will . . ." is not included in the statement. Discuss your findings with your classmates.

1. During this shift the patient will make a week's menu for new diabetic diet after reading instructions.
2. The patient will understand the importance of adhering to an exercise program after an explanation.
3. Encourage expression of anxiety this morning.
4. Discuss today some alternative plans for care following discharge.
5. Verbalize details regarding stated dissatisfaction with care given.

INTERVIEWS

Definition

The term "interview" tends to have different meanings. Some regard any goal—directed nurse-patient interaction as an interview. These persons view any interaction initiated for a purpose with a specified area of content to be an interview. Others tend to restrict the area of interviews to the application of information-gathering techniques in nurse-patient interactions.

Regardless of the differences in the meaning of the word "interview," most seem to agree that the interviewer is the primary information gatherer and the interviewee is the primary information giver. As related to nurse-patient communication, an interview will be considered to be a formal or informal interaction between patient and nurse (or other health care personnel) conducted primarily at the cognitive level for the purpose of obtaining specific information related to care of the patient.

This places many goal—directed nurse-patient interactions outside the scope of interviews. Communication for the purpose of establishing relationships, communication initiated to encourage the patient to verbalize feelings, and patient teaching are not grouped within the bounds of an interview, even though all are goal directed.

Parameters

Some type of relationship must be established if any communication is to be effective. It may consist of a friendly introduction with an explanation of the interview. The purpose is to inform the person being interviewed of the context of the forthcoming interaction. Patients expect questions to be asked during any hospitalization, but there are times unfortunately, when patients express annoyance because the same questions are repeated. The effective communicator is able to set the stage for an information-gathering interview without causing the patient any concern.

The interview is considered to be the primary data-gathering technique utilized in patient care. The use of interviews is invaluable in obtaining information on admission assessments, health histories, and nursing histories. Closed-ended questions are considered to be blocks to communication but are a necessary component in data collection. This does not exclude the use of open-ended questions but accepts closed-ended questions used to obtain specific pieces of data.

As indicated in the discussion of formal communication, notes may be made during the interview, since precise information is required for accurate assessments. For example, most institutions have forms to be completed during the admission interview. Much of the information can be obtained in a less formal way, but direct questioning obtains the most information in the shortest length of time. All too often the time factor is an element to be considered.

All interviews should be conducted in private. Much information directly related to the care of the patient is of a highly personal nature that the patient does not want to share with others. If privacy is not possible physically, a type of psychological privacy may be developed. Moving close to the patient and lowering the voice tends to exclude others who may be present, especially if backs are turned to them. The patient must be assured that any information given will be held in confidence. A professional attitude displayed by the nurse will convey this, and it can also be reinforced verbally.

Applications

The admission interview is usually a structured type of communication with specific items of information that must be elicited. The effective communicator will obtain much more information than what is included on the average admission form. These forms focus on physiological aspects; the nurse is concerned with psychological aspects as well.

The nurse is usually responsible for obtaining a health history. This is best obtained by use of interview techniques, whether formal or informal. Sometimes it is better accomplished in a more informal fashion. For example, in collecting data related to the current status and history of the current illness, open-ended questions may be more effective than closed-ended ones. By allowing the patient to take the lead in the interaction, the patient may volunteer information that is indirectly related to the current problem, information that the nurse would not have received with direct questioning.

In obtaining family and social histories, the nurse is often able to assess areas of concern that might have an impact on the patient's current status. The patient might express unpleasant feelings that have arisen during the course of the current illness, decisions that must be made, or problems aside from the current health problem that are a source of anxiety. Even though it would not be considered part of the interviewing process, the nurse can encourage verbalization of concerns. This can have a positive effect in enabling the patient to better cope with the current illness.

Interviews are always goal directed. They may be formal or informal. The approach used will vary with the interviewer and the situation. Some people are more comfortable using a structured format to obtain information, while others prefer an unstructured approach. Also, assessment of the patient will help in determining the type of interview to use since patients differ in their responsiveness to different approaches. The particular data desired may dictate the degree of formality of the interview.

CHECK IT OUT

Work in pairs to simulate an interview situation. The interviewee has complete freedom in fabricating answers. The interviewer is a nurse completing a health history. Information on the following is needed:
1. Childhood diseases
2. Past surgeries
3. Serious illnesses
4. Past hospitalizations
5. Last medical checkup
6. Current illness
7. Signs and symptoms
8. Current medications

The interviewer should use a formal approach on the first four items, asking for specific information on past health problems if desired. An informal approach should be used on the last four items to obtain data needed. Then change roles; use an informal approach on the first half and formal on the last.

Which approach did you prefer as an interviewer?
Which was more comfortable for the interviewee?

COMMUNICATING IN SPECIAL SITUATIONS

The preceding discussion of communication has been directed primarily toward the average adult patient. In the following pages, communication with patients in different age groups, such as children, teenagers, and the elderly, as well as patients who are visually impaired, hearing impaired, terminally ill, dysphasic, speaking a foreign language, or unable to read is discussed.

Communicating with Children and Teenagers

Children are not small adults. Their wants, needs, thinking processes, and emotional and physical status differ from that of an adult. Children's responses to communication approaches also will vary at different ages. Children often view hospitalization differently than an adult would. They may see it as a punishment, not as a means of getting well. Parents may inadvertently implant this idea with such statements as, "If you play out in the rain, you will get sick and have to go to the hospital."

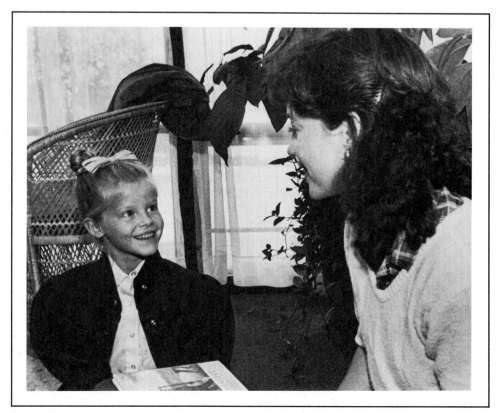

Regardless of the age of the child, each child should be treated as an individual with unique characteristics. The infant less than two years of age is often considered to be unaware of surroundings and somewhat unresponsive to others. This is not true. From the time of birth infants respond to paralanguage and to nonverbal communication such as touch. Establishing trust with the two-year-old child is important. This means being honest in any explanations; the child should be told if a procedure will hurt. Any explanation should be simple. For example, the application of a cast could be explained by saying, "You will go to sleep and wake up with a white stocking on your leg."

The four-year-old child wants to be independent but realizes that this is impossible. Consequently the child often becomes frustrated with the situation. This is an age in which children have a need for activity but want to do things their way. The nurse who is an effective communicator can enlist their cooperation by asking them to do things such as walk down the hall to get the breakfast tray or take the medicine cup to drink their medication. Praise and rewards are important at this age. Rewards may be in the form of mementos of the hospital stay, such as a syringe without a needle, medicine cups, or a badge saying, "Johnny is a good patient." The use of games may be effective. For example, the child can give an injection to a doll with a needleless syringe to make the doll well. Children in this age group need to be able to make choices, but only two alternatives should be presented, for example, "Would you like potatoes or rice with lunch?" or "Do you want to take a bath before or after breakfast?" Four-year-old children may ask open-ended questions such as "Why do I have to take this nasty medicine?" but want closed-ended answers. They do not want to know anything about the action of the medicine or the symptoms it will relieve, but only that it will make them well or that it will make it possible for them to go home sooner.

During the early school years, the child has a need for recognition and tends to be cooperative in striving to meet expectations. Since most children in this age group can deal with abstractions, communication can be at a more adult level. Words used should still be simple, but explanations can be more detailed than with younger children. Children in this age group are sensitive to criticism and will respond more positively to statements such as, "You hardly cried at all with that shot. You are real brave," than to "You are being a crybaby. That was just a little shot." During this age period, children identify closely with parents. Questions regarding how things are done at home are very effective. If the child describes a bedtime routine that involves the parents, it is helpful if the nurse can simulate the ritual in the hospital.

The preadolescent years are a time in which skills are developing and teamwork is an important aspect of the child's life. This is usually one of the most delightful age groups with which to work. Most preadolescents have retained the desire to please and have developed sufficient skills to be capable of many tasks. Since teamwork is important to them, the nurse can capitalize on this by explaining how the health team works together and enlist the child as a member of the team. These children feel more grown-up and cooperate more fully in their care if given the responsibility of tasks such as writing down the amount of fluids they have taken and the number of times and how far they have walked in the hall. This depends, of course, on the mental and physical ability of the child. The nurse may even make a list of medications and times for the child to mark off. Even though the nurse is keeping a record of everything, the child feels the responsibility of having a part in the care and will respond positively in following the prescribed regimen.

The primary complaint of hospitalized adolescents is that they are treated like a child. If admitted to a pediatric unit, the grievance is amplified. Adolescents want to be dealt with as adults; they want frank explanations from medical personnel. This is an age when the individual enjoys impressing peers with knowledge obtained from outside the classroom. The nurse can establish rapport with adolescents by treating them as adults with full explanations of their condition and treatment. They should be familiarized with medical terms. Drawings can be used to explain facts. The spelling, pronunciation, and meaning of unfamiliar medical terms can be explained to them. They often appreciate mementos of their hospitalization, such as a wisdom tooth that was removed or a disposable suture removal set. Empty intravenous solution containers and tubing can be used to make hummingbird feeders. These items, along with medical knowledge, are certain to impress their peers. The nurse should notice and express approval (or at least acceptance) of their teenage visitors. Adolescents who are able can be asked to talk to a lonely patient in the lounge or to entertain some of the younger children in the playroom. Careful assessments by the nurse are essential in making these requests.

The preceding discussion of approaches to and communication with children and teenagers is in general terms. Each child is unique and must be considered on an individual basis. Children are human beings and should have the rights and privileges corresponding to their level of development.

Communicating with Elderly Persons

As the percentage of elderly persons in the population increases, older patients comprise a greater percentage of patients in the hospital. Nurses must be aware that age is not the only factor to be considered; 70 years of age can be quite young for an active individual. Ageism has been noted as a rather prominent prejudice in our society; it is more pronounced in persons who have little knowledge of geriatrics or who have not experienced the benefits of companionship with an elderly person. Too often the nurse's image of an elderly person is that of a confused, tottering individual who needs total care. This may be true in some cases but is far from universal. Through awareness, experience, and education, attitudes toward the elderly can become more realistic and elderly persons' acceptance as individuals with special needs can become a prime consideration in assessments.

While it is true that elderly persons are individuals with different needs, it is also true that certain physiological changes occur with aging. There is a decreasing acuity of the senses, and reaction times are slowed. These factors have an impact on communication.

Elderly persons are rational adults who deserve a measure of respect. Regardless of their physical status, they should be treated as adults and not talked down to as if they were children. The nurse should always address them formally, for example, Mr. Brown or Mrs. Black, and not use the first name unless the patient has given permission to do so. This helps elderly patients to maintain their dignity. Patients will, however, frequently tell the nurse to call them by their first name, especially if the hospitalization is lengthy. Elderly persons will usually respond to requests made in a polite fashion more readily than to brusque directives. "Would you like to sit up to take these tablets?" will result in a more cooperative effort than, "Sit up and take your pills." (This should actually hold true for persons in any age group.) Any activity may take longer for an elderly person than for a younger person, verbal responses as well as physical activity. Patience is essential.

Elderly patients may become depressed when hospitalized. Their usual routines are disrupted, there may be a fear that this illness is the final one, they may miss visiting with neighbors, or they may worry about the spouse who is unable to visit frequently. Careful assessment is necessary to determine whether the symptoms are those of depression or signs that normally accompany aging, such as slowed speech, poor appetite, difficulty in concentrating, and reduced activity. If the patient is depressed, the nurse can help to improve the patient's frame of mind.

Any myth that elderly people have lost all traces of physical attractiveness must be dispelled. The patient's appearance—hair, complexion, make-up, after shave, or clothing—can be complimented. Telling older people how enjoyable it is to talk with them and letting them know that their viewpoint is respected can raise their self-esteem. This can improve self-motivation toward full cooperation in the therapeutic regimen.

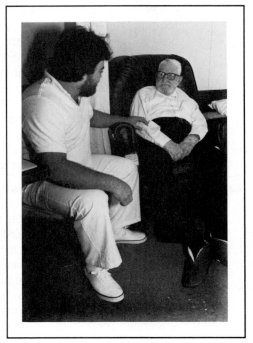

Most elderly persons are interested in current events. Many prefer the newspaper to television since it allows them to reread any item that is unclear. Hearing loss may also be a factor in watching television. Elderly persons, like persons of most age groups, are interested in and involved with the lives of their family and friends. Nurses who introduce themselves to the elderly patient's visitors and inquire about them later can establish a close relationship with the patient.

Elderly persons may take longer to process information. When procedures are scheduled, it is helpful to explain them well ahead of time. The patient should be given time to digest the information. The nurse should check later to see if there are any questions and repeat the information if necessary. The better the patient understands what is being done, the more cooperative that patient will be.

All elderly persons are aware that more of their life is behind them than in front of them. While everyone should be encouraged to live in the present, a life review—a review of what has happened in the past—may help the elderly to cope with the present. Reminiscing about past events can be enjoyable at any age. As a person becomes older there is more to reminisce about because of the number of years involved. Life review is not a matter of living in the past but a remembrance of all of the events that have led to the current stage in life. Recalling the past can help elderly persons to realize how full their life has been and enable them to accept the current situation, even though they may not have chosen it. If a person is hospitalized for a long period of time, finding someone such as a member of the family, a friend, or a volunteer to make notes of the events recalled by the patient can be a treasure for the family as well as serve as a stimulus for the patient.

In caring for and communicating with elderly patients, it must be kept in mind that they are individuals. Each one has different wants and needs, each brings a different frame of reference to the current situation, and each one is a unique human being. It is no more possible to stereotype the elderly person than it is to consider college students equal in all aspects.

CHECK IT OUT

In a small group select two students to be a nurse and a patient. Select one of the following patient roles for a nurse-patient interaction. At the end of the interaction have observers evaluate the responses of the nurse, noting effective techniques and suggesting any possible alternatives.

1. A 7-year-old child who does not want to go to bed.
2. A 14-year-old adolescent on a pediatric unit who complains that "The nurses treat me like a child."
3. A 72-year-old patient who is to be ambulated for the first time following knee surgery.

If there is time, select other students to perform other skits.

Communicating with Visually Impaired Patients

Although persons who are blind can hear the verbal part of communication, they are obviously unable to see nonverbal clues. The impact of nonverbal clues has been discussed at length in the preceding chapter. Interpretation of another person's communication may rely more on the nonverbal than the verbal message. Paralanguage is within the realm of reception, but facial expressions, body language, and gestures are not available for these persons. The sightless person's communication may be compared to talking on the telephone. It is true that telephone conversations are more effective than written letters for unimpaired persons, but face-to-face communication is usually preferred. When people say, "Great to see you looking so good," a blind person may have questions such as, "Do they mean it?", "Are they smiling?", or "Are they making fun of the way I'm dressed?"

Blindness imposes obstacles to communication for both receiver and sender. The sightless person tends to speak only when spoken to because of uncertainty of the presence and location of the other person or persons. Gesturing is limited and wide gestures avoided for fear of knocking something over. If several persons are in the room, speech may be loud because the sightless person is uncertain of the location of others. Any silence tends to make blind persons uncomfortable since they are unable to tell if others are present in the room.

The nurse customarily orients patients to the hospital's physical setting. Orientation of the blind patient must include an explanation of hospital sounds. Strange sounds can be frightening if the source is unknown. The orientation includes the physical setting with warnings of possible environmental obstacles. It is important to help all patients become or remain independent. This is especially true for blind patients. Patients who have recently lost their sight must replace skills lost as a result of loss of sight. Meals may be a particular problem. The clock placement of food on the tray with a description of the food accompanied by guided movements of the hands to locate each item is helpful. Privacy must be provided for practice.

Maintaining normal speech is a factor that will make the blind person more comfortable. The conscious avoidance of "sight" words and phrases, such as "Do you see what I mean?" or "Watch your step," is not necessary. These expressions have always been a part of the speech of persons who have recently lost their sight, and persons who have been sightless for a period of time have learned to accept them, often finding them amusing.

In communicating with a patient who is blind, it is very important for nurses to speak and identify themselves when entering the room, even though they might have just left the room. All procedures should be explained, with each step and its accompanying touch described. Touch is as important to a blind person as to a sighted person, but blind persons are not in need of constant touch. Nurses should attempt to put themselves in the patient's place and react with the patient as they would like others to react to them.

Communicating with Hearing Impaired Patients

Hearing loss may be as devastating as loss of vision. The person who is totally deaf tends to feel an aloneness as acute as that of the blind person. Deaf persons often exhibit a degree of paranoia, constantly looking over a shoulder because they are unable to hear if anything is behind them. Sounds and vibrations give life a dynamic quality. Sounds of nature can convey a sense of peace that cannot be derived from sight.

Deaf persons can communicate by sign language, but few hearing persons are able to use or understand sign language. One type of signing that is simple to learn is called finger spelling, in which letters are formed with one hand. This type of communication is very slow and tedious. Writing may be a simpler method of communicating with the hearing impaired than finger spelling. Many deaf persons are able to speechread. This was formerly called lip reading. The name was changed because the entire mouth and jaw are observed in the interpretation. This is only partially effective, however, since many words look the same but sound different.

Learning to communicate with a deaf patient requires patience and time on the part of both participants. Facing the patient with adequate light on the speaker's face is essential in speechreading. Speech must be slow and deliberate, with slightly exaggerated formation of words. Gesturing to the point of pantomime is sometimes effective.

Deaf patients may become stubborn and even hostile out of sheer frustration in trying to understand what is expected of them. Any time the nurse enters the room, a light touch on the arm will alert the patient to the nurse's presence. This is important because of the deaf person's tendency to be paranoiac. A person would be upset to look up and find a nurse about to give an injection when unaware that anyone was in the room.

Deaf persons do have the mechanisms for speech, and many learn to speak. Since they are unable to hear themselves, their speech often tends to be either a soft monotone or hollow and loud. Their frustration, however, comes more from trying to understand others than from trying to make themselves understood.

Communicating with Terminally Ill Patients

Death is an inescapable part of life, but a part that the average individual does not want to discuss. People often try to find an analogy for death, such as a crossing over, a meeting of loved ones who have passed, or an eternal rest. Terms such as these are frequently used to avoid saying that a loved one has died. The element of the unknown is probably the basis for the fear of death. No living person can say with certainty what occurs after death, even though non-Christians as well as Christians have beliefs related to happenings after death.

Various cultures view impending death from different perspectives. Some black persons and Mexican-Americans prefer being with the dying person, while persons of other cultures such as some Japanese-Americans do not. The American Indian has traditionally preferred dying alone. Anglo-Americans tend to be less in contact with death than many other cultures. Southeast Asians have many traditions regarding death but may have had to distance themselves from some in this country. This tends to extend the grieving process. The nurse should determine if the terminal patient wants to talk with a priest or other religious leader and make any contacts necessary. These are generalities regarding cultural views of death. It cannot be overemphasized that there are individual differences within each culture. These should be determined and respected.

Denial is often used by patients, family, and nurses when death is near. If the patient is using denial to cope with impending death, the nurse should not attempt to force the issue. There should be, however, a willingness to participate in any communication regarding death that is initiated by the patient. Health personnel tend to view death as defeat; they believe that their role is of a healing nature, of helping patients to progress from illness to wellness. When this does not happen the health care provider may feel that all efforts have been worthless.

Too often persons are hesitant to communicate with the terminally ill patient. Some say nothing for fear they might say the wrong thing. They fear that a remark might cause the patient more pain. The nurse may believe that nothing can be done about the situation so it is better not to talk about it. Family and friends tend to avoid visiting the dying patient for some of the same reasons the nurse avoids discussing death. When visitors are in the room, voices are hushed. The hesitancy to talk is linked to the fear of death felt by the living.

The dying person needs to be able to talk to others in order to express fears and to experience a closeness with loved ones. The isolation imposed on the dying by health personnel as well as by family and friends often triggers hostility in the patient and a withdrawal that makes the patient's last hours even more devastating for all concerned. Family and friends should be encouraged to talk in normal tones to the dying patient, to speak of current events, and to let the patient know that someone cares. Encouraging family to participate in care, such as wiping perspiration from the brow, applying ointment to dry lips, and applying lotion to arms may help the patient's family accept the death more readily. Nurses should not stay away from the room in this situation but should drop in often to see and check on the family as well as the patient, to offer coffee, and to talk with all present.

Terminally ill patients have the right to competent physical care and to be free of pain while receiving this care. They have the right to maintain their individuality as long as they are conscious and to have decisions respected even when contrary to the beliefs of others. Comatose patients are individuals and should be acknowledged as such. They should be talked to directly. Their condition should never be discussed in their presence; persons in the room should assume that the patient can still hear. No patient should be allowed to die alone. This right should receive top priority. The terminally patient has a right to satisfying communication with others. Too often social conversation and standard responses are used to avoid any serious conversation about death and dying. However, dying persons often want to talk about feelings. Effective communicators can help the patient discuss concerns about death and feel more at peace with the world. They can help the family say goodbye to the patient. This benefits both patient and family.

The terminally ill patient may need help in various areas such as business affairs, wills, and funeral details. While the nurse cannot take care of all of these details, contacting those who can helps put the patient's mind at ease. Sometimes the nurse is the only person with whom the patient can communicate. Any mention of death may bring forth tears in family and friends. Watching a loved one die is not easy, but the dying person who is deserted by loved ones faces a much more difficult task. The nurse must let dying patients know that they will not be left alone.

The nurse must be prepared to discuss whatever topic the patient introduces. Some terminally ill patients may fantasize and plan lengthy trips or new occupations. The nurse needs to know the patient well in responding to these fantasies. Some patients can accept death and inject a bit of humor into the situation. Whatever the patient's approach to the subject of death, the nurse's attitude needs to be one of acceptance.

Dying patients need to be allowed to make choices and to remain in control as much as possible. The nurse should show them alternatives available. For example, if a patient wants to die at home, the help available should be discussed and any necessary arrangements should be made. All questions should be answered honestly, but information that is not requested need not be volunteered. Nurses may say they do not have time to talk with patients, but the dying patient has less time than the nurse. Families may be harder to deal with than the patient in some instances. The nurse should listen to all they have to say. Some issues are better resolved before death; the nurse can help the patient and family discuss them together. The family's participation in care as mentioned previously may be helpful. Articles that are meaningful to the patient for sharing memories can be brought from home. Families can also keep a diary of what the patient talks about during the last days. This can be a comfort when the loved one is no longer with them.

Dying patients need to know that others care about them as individuals. The nurse expresses care through communication. Caring for a dying patient is a risk. The nurse may experience grief and loss because of risking a feeling of love and attachment for the patient. However, most nurses will say it was well worth it.

Communicating with Patients Who Are Dysphasic

Dysphasia is impairment of speech resulting from a brain lesion. The term aphasia usually indicates absence (but sometimes includes impairment) of ability to communicate related to dysfunction of brain centers. These disorders are frequently seen as the result of a stroke. Difficulty in speaking may be caused by neurological disorders such as Parkinson's disease. Dysarthria is caused by a dysfunction of the muscles involved in speech rather than by a brain lesion. Both dysphasia and dysarthria create communication problems for the individual. Inability to communicate isolates a person from the world. Friends may no longer visit since they think the person no longer recognizes them since there is limited or no communication. Dysarthria makes speech slow, difficult, and hard to understand. Friends may not have the patience to try to carry on a conversation with individuals with this disorder.

The dysphasic person may have difficulties in decoding messages, but the primary problem is in the encoding. A wide range of devices is available to help these patients. The simplest is the letter, word, or picture board. These are available in many hospitals, but they can be constructed easily if they are not available. Pictures of various activities can be used to determine the patient's wishes, for example, a meal on a tray to denote hunger, a glass to indicate thirst, or a bedpan or bathroom. A word chart with words frequently used to make requests or to express satisfaction facilitates communication. A letter board can be used if the patient is able to spell. There are many computer-assisted devices such as scanners that allow the patient to stop at appropriate responses. Messages may be transmitted on a computer or on a magic slate if the patient is able to utilize these aids. These methods are good interim devices, but the primary aim is to restore normal speech if at all possible.

It is difficult to put oneself in the dysphasic patient's place and to know how it feels to be unable to communicate one's thoughts. The blocking of speech produces extreme frustration and a feeling of helplessness. Early treatment before the patient gives up hope and becomes depressed is imperative. If an avenue of communication is not established, hostility and anger will inevitably follow. This will inhibit progress in other areas of rehabilitation, since the patient will often resist all treatment. Finding some method of communication will not only lessen the sense of isolation but will give a sense of hope and self-esteem. Communication is such a great part of a person's self-identity that impairment brings a feeling of loss of self.

Communicating with Patients Who Speak Foreign Languages

How can a person communicate with another who speaks a different language? Since it seems unlikely that there will be a universal language in the foreseeable future and since populations are increasingly mobile, this is a problem worth consideration. An interpreter is the obvious answer, but this poses some difficulties. Communication can be misconstrued by an interpreter who is not trained in the medical field. Hospitals in areas in which there are a number of foreign speaking people should and often do have trained interpreters in full-time positions.

With trained interpreters, nurses are able to communicate more effectively. Using short units of speech and waiting for a response simplifies obtaining the desired information; this gives an example for the patient to follow. Sometimes the summary approach is used in translating. This can be effective in such areas as explaining hospital routines but should be limited to the commonalities in information giving and receiving. Nonverbal behaviors always enhance communication. The more the nurse knows about different cultures, the more readily the nonverbal behaviors can be assessed. An understanding of the cultural differences also enables the nurse to be able to phrase questions properly. Much of the responsibility in the phrasing will lie with the interpreter, but the knowledgeable nurse is better able to direct the interpreter.

The nurse should keep medical terms to a minimum when messages must be translated, just as a knowledgeable interpreter should minimize any jargon of the patient or translate it into terms understood by the nurse. Patients from some cultures may introduce rambling accounts into what should be a short answer in response to a question. This may be related to their background of folk medicine in which factors often considered irrelevant are closely tied to beliefs about health. There are still many places in which folk medicine is the primary health care source. A fast diagnosis and quick cure (or promise of such) is expected. Fear on the part of the patient who is unfamiliar with the language and many other details of a medical facility may disrupt communication.

Sometimes the family or friends of the patient are recruited to act as an interpreter. This should be done as only a last resort. Communication through a third party is always difficult. The nurse must maintain rapport with the interpreter as well as with the patient and family to effectively communicate and care for the patient who speaks a foreign language.

Communicating with Patients Who Are Unable to Read

It may seem surprising that in a country with compulsory education there are well over 20 million people who cannot read, but it is a fact. Inability to read does not mean that a person cannot recognize some words and understand basic reading material at an elementary level. Functional illiteracy means that a majority of words will be recognized but only a small percentage understood. People with this problem are not always from lower economic classes. Some self-made business persons are able to memorize sufficient information to succeed.

How does a nurse determine if a patient is unable to read? There are many clues that the nurse can observe in order to assess reading ability. When patients are given a menu to select a diet, do they ask the nurse to fill it out or state that they do not care what is on it? Or is the selection a strange one? If the patient is given literature to read, are reading glasses misplaced? The nurse should compare the amount of information retained from oral instructions and written instructions. If a patient asks questions regarding a self-explanatory instruction sheet, this usually indicates a reading difficulty.

When the nurse has determined that a patient cannot read, what can be done? The hospital is not the environment for teaching reading, but the patient can be referred to an adult basic education course. The nurse can use drawings to illustrate things the patient is to do or refrain from doing. Any procedures can be explained in detail with the patient repeating the instructions. Patience is a key factor in helping the patient to understand what is expected; the nurse's patience will be rewarded when the patient understands what is happening and is able to cooperate fully in care.

VERBATIM RECORDING OF NURSE-PATIENT INTERACTIONS

Recordings of nurse-patient interactions are not intended as an additional tool in assessing the physical status of the patient. They are a tool for the nurse to use in learning communication skills. The recording should reflect the use of effective communication techniques to encourage the patient to verbalize. Many questions will be directed toward the affective level as the patient communicates anxieties and misunderstandings. Others will tend toward the cognitive level as solutions to problems are sought. These recordings should be as helpful to the student as to the instructor in evaluating communication ability. Students can evaluate their own approach to communication and pinpoint weaknesses, thus improving communication effectiveness. Communication strengths should be noted to gain an appreciation of approaches and techniques that are truly facilitative.

Planning a Nurse-Patient Communication Interaction

Communication is sometimes more effective if a measure of planning is involved. Planning may include making an appointment with the patient. This is usually done in a very informal manner such as, "I'll be back after you have had a chance to rest and we can talk." When there is an opportunity to plan, the nurse can take into account factors noted in environmental management to make the setting more conducive to communication. Time can be planned when there will be the least amount of interruptions and the readiness of both participants is maximum. This is especially important in relation to the patient. Assessment of level of energy and physical comfort is the major determinant.

Components of a Verbatim Recording

The format presented is suggested as a method of recording a nurse-patient communication interaction. The setting and goal are taken into consideration to present a more complete overall picture. The patient's and the nurse's nonverbal as well as verbal messages are recorded. Each response used by the nurse is identified as a specific facilitator or block and evaluated. The components will be discussed separately to indicate the information to be included in each column of the form.

Setting

The setting is included to give an insight into any environmental factors that may have helped or hindered the interaction. This may include the time of day and any activities taking place as well as the physical setting.

Goal

The goal does not have to be planned in writing nor must it remain static. Often there will not be a goal until the patient indicates the need to communicate a concern. This is the point at which the effective communicator follows through on the cue given by the patient. The nurse may intend to discuss certain aspects of an illness but may pick up on a cue that determines the general direction of the remainder of the interaction. When recording an interaction, the goal should be stated relative to the interaction, whether planned ahead or spontaneously formulated in response to a cue.

Verbal Communication

The verbal component, the recording of what each participant says, is the substance of any interaction. The responses of each participant must be clearly indicated in the first column on the form. Notes should not be taken during this process since this would detract from the spontaneity. However, notes should be made as soon as possible to retain the wording as closely as possible.

Nonverbal Communication

Including the nonverbal component gives a better perspective of the situation for review. It enhances the evaluation of the recording, since nonverbal behaviors may convey as much as or more than the verbal message. Paralanguage as well as facial expressions, gestures, and body language in general should be a part of this component.

Technique

The nurse's technique is identified. No techniques are noted for the patient since the purpose is not to evaluate the patient's ability to communicate effectively. The nurse is the participant in the interaction who is encouraging communication and helping the patient to express feelings or consider alternative solutions to a problem. There may be blocks used by the nurse. These should be noted even though blocks do not always interrupt the course of communication. Techniques should be labeled according to the terms used in this text to avoid confusion.

Evaluation

The evaluation is of the nurse's responses and the application of facilitative communication techniques. If the response was considered a block, this fact should be stated and a notation made of a facilitative technique that could have been used. If a facilitative technique was used but an alternative one would have been more effective, the preferred response should be noted. If the facilitator was effective in encouraging communication, this should be reflected in the recording. The positive should be emphasized, rather than dwelling on the negative. The student nurse is not expected to perform to perfection in communicating with the patients. Even experienced nurses often fail to see the most effective methods.

Example of a Nurse-Patient Communication Interaction

Figure 4-1, a verbatim recording of a nurse-patient communication interaction, shows the type of information to be included in each column. The techniques used are not all facilitative. Those that are not facilitative have an evaluation with possible alternatives. This is not meant to be a complete nurse-patient interaction but to serve as an illustration of the beginning of a meaningful interchange. These verbatim recordings are not meant to give an account of a casual introduction or social conversation. They are not intended to note the manner in which the nurse explained that it was time for a certain procedure and the manner in which the procedure would be accomplished. Nor are they intended to record instructions given to the patient. While explanations to the patient and patient teaching are of prime importance, the recording of a nurse-patient interaction should reflect therapeutic communication with an expression of feelings by the patient or the search for solutions to problems.

NURSE-PATIENT COMMUNICATION INTERACTION

SETTING: Patient's private room before A.M. care

GOAL: Verbalize concerns regarding possible diagnosis. (Goal not formulated until patient expressed concern.)

| SENDER | COMMUNICATION | | TECHNIQUE | EVALUATION |
	VERBAL	NONVERBAL		
S.N.	Good morning, Mrs. N. Are you feeling better this morning?	Standing by bed	Closed-ended question	Should be open-ended— How are you feeling?
Mrs. N.	No. I didn't sleep last night.	Frowning		
S.N.	Didn't sleep?	Holding hand	Reflection	To encourage details
Mrs. N.	No. Those night nurses won't do anything.	Glaring at S.N.		
S.N.	The night nurses on this unit are usually very good.	Stepping back from bed	Defending	Bad block. Should have asked what happened
Mrs. N.	They weren't last night. I'd go home now if I could.	Raising up on elbow; biting lip		
S.N.	You seem very upset.	Moving back to bed	Validating	To check interpretation
Mrs. N.	Wouldn't you be? I'm afraid I have cancer.	Eyes watery		
S.N.	I'm sure I'd be very concerned. I have plenty of time if you would like to talk about it.	Sitting by bed, holding hand	Acknowledging feelings; open-ended statement	To encourage verbalization

Figure 4.1 Nurse-patient communication interaction.

The length of the interaction is not an important criterion; some short interchanges are more therapeutic than longer ones. The patient's name should never appear on these forms as this could be construed as a disclosure of privileged information. Students should put their knowledge of communication techniques into action and record their progress as effective communicators.

IN A CAPSULE

The *affective level* of communication is the feeling or emotional component, while the *cognitive* level is based on factual information and reasoning. *Formal communication* is goal directed and structured to obtain the greatest amount of information in the shortest length of time. There is no definite structure in *informal communication*, even though there may be a goal. *Social communication* consists more of impersonal interchanges without a specific goal. *Goal-directed communication* is usually more effective when some planning is involved.

Communication *goals* reflect the end result to be achieved. Effective goals are *realistic*, *measurable*, *mutually acceptable*, and state a *time frame*. In nurse-patient relationships, the goal should be *patient centered* and may or may not be *written*. *Interviews* are primarily goal-directed interactions using a formal or an informal approach to obtain specified data.

Communicating with *the child* requires adaptation of techniques to meet the needs of the individuals within the age or developmental range. There are special considerations in communicating with the *elderly*, but each one is an individual who is unique in background and in current needs. Special approaches in communication are applied with *visually* and *hearing impaired patients*. The nurse needs to be prepared to communicate with the *terminally ill* patient on any topic of the patient's choosing. The blocking of speech in the *dysphasic* patient produces frustration, making communication an immediate concern. The nurse needs a trained interpreter plus an understanding of cultural differences to effectively communicate with the patient who speaks a *foreign language*. Illustrations, patience, and understanding are required for communication with the patient who is *unable to read*.

Verbatim recordings of *nurse-patient communication interactions* serve as a tool for evaluation of communication effectiveness. They should include *nonverbal* as well as *verbal* communication with an *evaluation* of the *technique* used. Notation of the *setting* of the interaction and the *goal* make the record more complete.

DO YOU REMEMBER

- the difference in affective and cognitive levels of communication?
- considerations in planning goal-directed communication?
- uses of interviews in nurse-patient communication?
- special approaches in communication with visually and hearing impaired patients?
- the frustration felt by dysphasic patients and methods to establish communication with them?

- pertinent points in communicating with patients who speak foreign languages?
- responsibilities of the nurse when the patient is unable to read?
- the components of a nurse-patient interaction recording?

CAN YOU DESCRIBE

- formal and informal communication?
- the application of social communication in the health care setting?
- the format of an effective goal?
- various techniques that are considered more effective with children in different age groups?
- approaches that enhance the effectiveness of communication with the elderly?
- responsibilities of the nurse in communicating with the terminally ill?
- the purpose of verbatim recordings of nurse-patient communication?

ACTION, PLEASE

1. What is it like to be blind?

    a. Take time to experience the world of the sightless. With a friend or a family member, take turns at being blind. Place a blindfold securely over your eyes. Have the sighted participant lead the blind person around outdoors, go up or down stairs, warn of any obstacles, and allow the "blind" person to brush against something that is not potentially harmful.

    b. Trade places and repeat. What were your reactions when blindfolded? How dependent did you feel? What was your response to a strange noise? How important is it for you to identify yourself when entering a blind patient's room?

_____

_____

_____

_____

_____

_____

    c. If you want to gain further insights, eat a meal blindfolded.

2. Complete a nurse-patient communication interaction on a form similar to Figure 4-1. Have two classmates critique the recording.

3. *How would you respond?* You are assigned to care for Miss Goines, a 36-year-old woman with a brain abscess who has not responded to medical or surgical treatment. While you are caring for her she says, "I need someone to help me plan my funeral service so it won't be a problem for my family when I die."

a. What would your initial emotional response be?

_____

_____

b. Could you discuss her request with her?

_____

_____

c. How would you convey the idea that you understand and are willing to listen?

_____

_____

_____

d. Would you contact the hospital chaplain or her minister to relieve you of the responsibility? State your reasons.

_____

_____

_____

There is no right or wrong answer in this situation. It is not an unrealistic solution; you may be confronted with a similar situation. Discuss it with your classmates.

UNIT I BIBLIOGRAPHY

Atkinson, Leslie D., and Murray, Mary E. *Fundamentals of Nursing: A Nursing Process Approach.* New York: Macmillan Publishing Co., Inc., 1985.

Bernstein, Basil. Elaborated and restricted codes: Their social origins and some consequences. In A. G. Smith (Ed.), *Language and Poverty.* New York: Holt, Rinehart & Winston, 1966.

Bigelow-Kemp, Brenda and Pilliterri, Adele. *Fundamentals of Nursing: A Framework for Practice.* Boston: Little, Brown and Company, 1984.

Blondis, Marion N. and Jackson, Barbara E. *Nonverbal Communication with Patients.* New York: John Wiley & Sons, 1982.

Boyle, Joyceen S. and Andrews, Margaret M. *Transcultural Concepts in Nursing Care.* Glenview, Illinois: Scott, Foresman and Company, 1989.

Bradley, Jean C. and Edinberg, Mark A. *Communication in the Nursing Context.* Norwalk, Connecticut: Appleton-Century-Crofts, 1982.

Burgess, Ann Wolbert and Lazare, Aaron. *Psychiatric Nursing in the Hospital and the Community.* Second Edition. Englewood Cliffs, New Jersey: Prentice-Hall, Inc., 1973.

Carlson, Robert E., *The Nurse's Guide to Better Communication.* Glenview, Illinois: Scott, Foresman and Company, 1984.

Collins, Mattie. *Communication in Health Care.* Saint Louis: The C. V. Mosby Company, 1977.

Cormier, L. Sherilyn, et al. *Interviewing and Helping Skills for Health Professionals.* Monterey, California: Wadsworth Health Sciences Division, 1984.

Craig, Grace J. *Human Development.* Englewood Cliffs, New Jersey: Prentice-Hall, Inc., 1976.

Crane, Alison L. Why Sickness Can Be a Laughing Matter. *RN*, February 1987, 41-42.

Dolan, Marion B. A Drug You Can't Overuse. *RN*, November, 1985, 47-48.

Duldt, Bonnie W., et al. *Interpersonal Communication in Nursing.* Philadelphia; F. A. Davis Company, 1984.

Ellis, Janice R. and Nowlis, Elizabeth A. *Nursing: A Human Needs Approach*, Third Edition. Boston: Houghton Mifflin Company, 1985.

Fritz, Paul A., et al. *Interpersonal Communication in Nursing.* Norwalk, Connecticut: Appleton-Century-Crofts, 1984.

Grace, Helen K., et al. *Mental Health Nursing: A SocioPsychological Approach.* Dubuque, Iowa: Wm. C. Brown Company Publishers, 1977.

Grasska, Merry Ann and McFarland, Teresa. Overcoming the Language Barrier: Problems and Solutions. *American Journal of Nursing*, September, 1982, 1376-1382.

Herth, Kaye A. Laughter, a Nursing Rx. *American Journal of Nursing*, August 1984, 991-992.

Klinzing, Dennis and Klinzing, Dene. *Communication for Allied Health Professionals.* Dubuque, Iowa: Wm. C. Brown Publishers, 1985.

Kozier, Barbara and Erb, Glenora. *Fundamentals of Nursing: Concepts and Procedures*, Third Edition. Menlo Park, California: Addison-Wesley Publishing Company, 1987.

Kumin, Libby and Rysticken, Noreen. Aids to Bridge the Communication Barrier. *Geriatric Nursing*, November/December, 1985, 348-351.

Long, Lynette and Prophit, Sister Penny. *Understanding/Responding.* Monterey, California: Wadsworth Health Sciences Division, 1981.

Loughrey, Linda. Dealing with the Illiterate Patient . . . You Can't Read Him Like a Book. *Nursing 83*, January, 1983, 65-67.

Manfreda, Marguerite L. *Psychiatric Nursing.* Philadelphia: F. A. Davis Company, 1975.

Narrow, Barbara W. and Buschle, Kay B. *Fundamentals of Nursing Practice*, Second Edition. New York: John Wiley & Sons, 1987.

Northouse, Peter G. and Northouse, Laurel L. *Health Communication.* Englewood Cliffs, New Jersey: Prentice-Hall, Inc., 1985.

Osterlund, Rob. Humor, A Serious Approach to Patient Care. *Nursing '83*, December 1983, 46-47.

Potter, Patricia A. and Perry, Anne G. *Fundamentals of Nursing: Concepts, Process, and Practice.* St. Louis: The C. V. Mosby Company, 1985.

Rice, Liz. Do We Discriminate Against the Elderly? *Nursing 88*, March, 1988, 44-45.

Robinson, Vera M. *Humor and the Health Professions.* Thorofare, New Jersey: Charles B. Slack, Inc., 1977.

Sathre, Freda S. et al. *Let's Talk,* Second Edition. Glenview, Illinois: Scott, Foresman and Company, 1977.

Smith, Voncile M. and Bass, Thelma M. *Communication for Health Professionals.* Philadelphia: J. B. Lippincott Company, 1979.

Sorensen, Karen C. and Luckmann, Joan. *Basic Nursing: A Psychophysiological Approach,* Second Edition. Philadelphia: W. B. Saunders Company, 1986.

Steele, Shirley M. and Harmon, Vera M. *Values Clarification in Nursing,* Second Edition. Norwalk, Connecticut: Appleton-Century-Crofts, 1983.

Weaver, Richard L. II. *Understanding Interpersonal Communication,* Fourth Edition. Glenview Illinois: Scott, Foresman and Company, 1987.

Wilson, Karen. I Learned About Life from Harry's Death. *RN,* April, 1987, 58-62.

Wolff, LuVerne et al. *Fundamentals of Nursing,* Seventh Edition. Philadelphia: J. B. Lippincott Company, 1983.

The Nurse As Patient/Family Teacher

CHAPTER

5

Fundamentals of the Teaching/ Learning Process

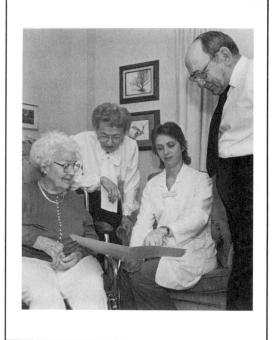

There is no substitute for accurate knowledge. **Randall Jacobs**

OBJECTIVES

Upon completion of this chapter, the student will be able to:

- identify the basic domains of learning.
- relate the significance of learning modes to patient teaching.
- state the manner in which at least eight of the factors noted enhance learning.
- discuss the relationship of physical or emotional stress to learning.
- note ways in which the nurse might inadvertently obstruct learning.
- identify five or more factors that contribute to the effectiveness of patient teaching.
- explain obstacles that might hinder patient teaching.
- describe the application of various teaching strategies.
- explain the use of adjuncts to teaching or teaching aids.

GLOSSARY OF TERMS*

Adjuncts to teaching   Added as an accompaniment in a secondary position.
Domains of learning   Spheres of influence or activity in the learning process.
  Cognitive domain   The learning of factual knowledge.
  Affective domain   Learning related to feelings or emotions.
  Psychomotor domain   Learning involving motor action proceeding from mental activity.
Learning   Modification of a behavioral tendency through experience.
Motivation   The provision of an incentive, a need or desire, to take action.
Programmed instruction   Instructional material with questions and answers interspersed throughout content designed for learner mastery without assistance.
Teaching strategy   A device or method for accomplishing a desired end in the teaching/learning process.

*Definitions applicable to content.

Patient teaching is one of the ways in which nurses communicate with patients, a form of goal-oriented communication. Nurses have always instructed patients in health matters as part of bedside care. Giving directions for care of infants, for oral hygiene, for applying dressings, for taking medications, and for many other aspects of health and hygiene has always been considered one of the duties of nurses.

However, teaching has not always been planned formally or documented carefully. These responsibilities are now seen in a more structured manner. One role of the nurse is that of patient/family teacher. The term "patient teaching" or "patient eduction" is generally accepted to mean "patient/family education." References to patient teaching or patient education throughout this unit include the family, even though not specifically stated each time.

In order to be an effective teacher, it is essential to understand the basic principles of teaching and learning. This chapter is an introduction to principles to be applied in patient teaching as a part of patient care. Through the application of the principles presented, students can develop their own approach to teaching.

CHARACTERISTICS OF LEARNING

Learning is not something that takes place before adulthood and then stops. It is a lifelong process. The use of the term "learning process" indicates that it is active and ongoing. True learning results in a more or less permanent change in behavior as a result of the experience. Adults, including the elderly, are capable of learning. The process may be slower in the later years, but learning does take place at all ages. Since individuals are complex creatures with varied behaviors and emotions, learning must be an individualized process. Each person learns in a particular way, and no one way is right for all.

Basic Domains of Learning

Learning takes place in different domains. The cognitive and affective domains were introduced in Unit I. These, as well as the psychomotor domain, are applicable to the teaching/learning process.

Cognitive Domain

The cognitive domain involves the thinking self. Learning too often is seen as limited to this domain. During the school years it may seem like only the thinking process is involved in learning. This is a significant part of all learning. Many of the aspects of patient teaching will be in the cognitive domain. Teaching about the pathophysiology of a disease or the reason for a certain treatment involves the thinking process. For example, teaching a patient about what happens in the body when a person has diabetes and why it is necessary to take insulin involves thinking or cognitive processes.

Affective Domain

Patient teaching involves the affective domain as well as the cognitive. The affective domain is the feeling part of the individual. Affective concepts are more difficult to convey to the patient and more difficult to evaluate, but they are a part of patient education. Learning to cope with physical limitations such as the necessity of using a walker for ambulation involves motor skills. However, the affective domain is also involved as the person accepts the reality of the situation. Concepts of feeling comfortable with breast-feeding a baby or giving oneself an insulin injection each day are part of affective learning.

Psychomotor Domain

The psychomotor domain involves motor activity. It is a visible and readily evaluated domain in patient teaching. The psychomotor domain includes skills that are necessary for the patient or family to provide adequate care after discharge. The skills to be taught range from simple skills, such as application of ointment to a specified area, to complex skills, such as irrigation and dressing of a wound or peritoneal dialysis. Regardless of the simplicity or complexity of the skills involved, it is important that the patient or family demonstrate competency in performance of essential skills prior to discharge.

Dietary education for a diabetic patient can illustrate the different domains applied to a single aspect of care. The cognitive domain might include the patient's selection of foods for a week to meet the stated criteria of the prescribed diet. In the psychomotor domain, the patient could prepare these foods for several days if facilities were available. The affective domain might concern the patient's acceptance of the diabetic diet in adhering to it after discharge. Each domain deals with one subject—the diabetic diet—but represents teaching/learning in its own way. Content to be taught cannot always be approached in all three domains.

Learning Modes

Learning is an individualized process. People do not all learn in the same manner. The approach chosen for learning is not linked to intelligence but is simply a matter of personal preference. The resulting knowledge can be the same regardless of the approach chosen.

Global versus Linear Learners

One manner in which learning is classified is global and linear. Some persons need to look at the overall picture first and then study the details. This approach to learning is often termed global. Others will take a linear approach, preferring to study each component of the picture before looking at the whole.

An example of this is the construction of a garment. A detailed set of instructions is always included in the pattern. The person who takes the global approach will look first at the picture of the finished garment and consider the steps later. The person who prefers the linear approach will follow the instructions step by step with little reference to the finished product. Both will end up with finished garments, but they will have approached the process differently.

Another example is nursing students learning to apply an Ace bandage. The global learner will look first at the appearance of the bandage after it is applied. The linear learner will follow the steps in the procedure from the first step, anchoring the bandage. The goal attained is the same for both, but the method of approach differs.

Visual Learners

Some individuals tend to be visual learners. Material is assimilated more readily by these persons when it is presented graphically. They are the students who can read a chapter in a text and be able to grasp the essential facts. These learners, however, do not follow verbal directions readily. They are usually very observant, the persons who can walk through a room and remember every detail of the furnishings. Verbal explanations need to be accompanied by visual representations for these learners to fully comprehend the material.

Auditory Learners

The auditory learner, or the other hand, can readily grasp verbal explanations. Oral directions are more readily comprehended by them than written instructions. Any graphic representations need to be accompanied by a verbal explanation to enhance their learning.

Kinesthetic Learners

Another type of learning is referred to as kinesthetic. The kinesthetic learner prefers an active learning process. This person needs demonstrations and the opportunity to repeat the performance observed. The student in nursing who is a kinesthetic learner tends to gain more from clinical experience than classroom discussion.

These are some representations of different modes of learning. Very few people are purely one type or another. Most people are a combination, with a tendency to prefer one mode to another. No particular mode is superior to another. The mode of learning is an individual factor that should be taken into account in planning any teaching. The explanations given are simplified but may help in planning patient teaching approaches. The teaching plan may be primarily in one mode or may encompass all of the modes. Having material available in more than one mode enables the plan to be adapted for multiple use.

GENERAL PRINCIPLES OF LEARNING

A person can read a dozen texts and find twelve different lists of principles of learning. One aspect may be emphasized in one list and missing from another. In the following paragraphs generally accepted principles that apply to all age groups are discussed. They are intended to give an overall picture of the learning process and to help in planning patient teaching. Figure 5-1 represents the application of principles in maximizing learning.

EFFECTIVE LEARNING

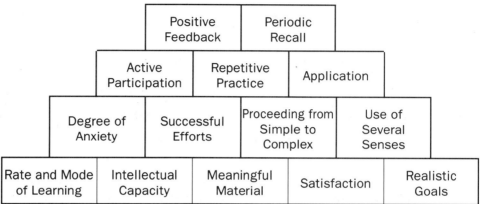

Figure 5.1: Building blocks of effective learning

Factors That Enhance Learning

Factors that enhance learning may be considered the positive aspects of learning. They are generally applicable to most situations. Many have been proven in various studies. These are factors that should be kept in mind when planning patient teaching. They include rate and mode of learning, intellectual capacity, meaningful material, satisfaction, realistic goals, degree of anxiety, successful efforts, proceeding from simple to complex, use of several senses, active participation, repetitive practice, application, positive feedback and periodic recall.

Rate and Mode of Learning

Individuals learn at their own speed and in their own way. The preferred mode and the rate of speed are variables in the learning process. Some individuals learn quickly but do not retain the material for a long period of time. Others are slower to learn but retain the material longer. This is not to say that fast learners do not retain information for a long period of time, but that learning patterns differ. It is a mistake to try to force one particular mode on the learner or to put a time frame on learning.

Intellectual Capacity

Intellectual capacity of the learner determines the amount that can be learned. Learning is not completely tied to intelligence, but some individuals are unable to progress beyond a certain point in learning. Some patients' capacity to learn may be limited, as in mental retardation. These patients can learn some things, but it is frustrating for both patient and nurse for the nurse to try to teach complicated procedures to persons who do not have the ability to grasp them.

Meaningful Material
The learner only learns things that are considered meaningful. This is an important principle to remember in planning patient teaching. Before presenting material it is essential to convince the patient of the usefulness of what is being taught.

Satisfaction
A feeling of satisfaction gained from the learning experience tends to prolong the length of retention of the material. If the learner feels that the material fulfills a need, the facts will be integrated into the individual's experience and retained for future reference.

Realistic Goals
Realistic goal setting is essential to learning. The expected outcome must be one the patient believes can be accomplished. If goals are set too high, failure often results, since the patient does not believe that it is possible to reach the goal. Some argue that goals set too low limit performance. However, small successes give the patient the incentive to accomplish the goal.

Degree of Anxiety
A degree of anxiety motivates the learner. This does not mean the extreme degree of anxiety that keeps a person from doing anything, but enough concern to strive to accomplish something. Patient adherence to a prescribed regimen is promoted by a moderate degree of anxiety. This is true in all learning. The person must feel a necessity to learn, which produces a degree of anxiety. Complete absence of anxiety results in complacency.

Successful Efforts
Success in learning promotes further success and better toleration of failure. No one wants to fail. The learner must be praised for small successes to realize that success in attaining the goal is possible. Difficulty can be accepted if previous efforts have been successful. For example, a nursing student may be learning to give injections. Inserting the needle into the model properly may be difficult for the student. However, the instructor may have complimented the student on withdrawing the exact amount into the syringe. The inability to insert the needle properly on the first attempt does not destroy the student's self-confidence because there was a previous success. Any success builds the learner's self-confidence and can act as a motivating factor in additional learning experiences.

Proceeding from Simple to Complex
Understanding is increased by proceeding from simple to complex. This is a basic principle that is easily recognized and applied. There may be some differences of opinion in the use of the terms "simple" and "complex." What is easy for one person may be difficult for another. A complex procedure can be broken down into a series of simple steps. In a nursing program, the simple procedures are introduced first. The average beginning student with no hospital experience would be overwhelmed if assigned to care for a patient on a respirator. However, the senior student is able to handle the complex procedures necessary to care for this patient because the simple tasks that make up this complex task have been previously mastered.

Use of Several Senses

Learning is increased when more than one of the senses is involved. Regardless of the mode of learning preferred by the learner, the more input through different senses, the more firmly the information is imprinted in the memory. In planning patient education, there may not be time to assess the preference of the learner for the mode of learning. If material is presented through two or more of the senses, the information should be well received, regardless of the patient's preference.

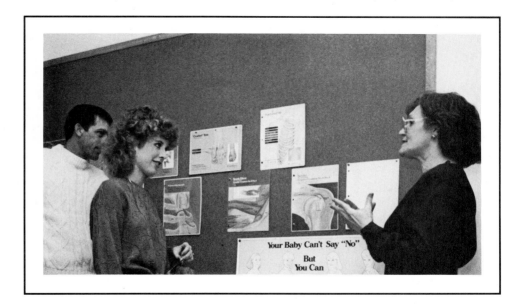

Active Participation

Active participation enhances learning. Students usually gain more from a class in which they ask questions and enter into a discussion than one in which they sit quietly and only listen. The patient also needs to be given an opportunity to ask questions and to express any concerns. Active participation in the planning as well as implementation of the subject to be learned will facilitate learning and increase retention.

Repetitive Practice

Repetitive practice is essential for learning skills. It would be very difficult to give an injection, for example, if the student had watched a demonstration but had not practiced or had tried it only once. Patients frequently require more practice than students in learning this type of skill since they will be on their own after discharge.

Application

The shorter the length of time from learning to application, the greater the amount of material retained. This is true of facts but especially skills. For example, a diabetic patient is taught about diet and insulin injection, but meals are served without comment and the nurses continue to give the insulin. After returning home, the patient is very unsure of the method of preparing and giving the insulin and must refer to the written diet list for all meals. Allowing patients to plan a diet and give injections prior to discharge will give them enough self-confidence to care for themselves after discharge.

Positive Feedback

Learning is enhanced by feedback from the instructor. This feedback is the evaluation of the learner's performance in meeting a specific goal. Patients need to be made aware of their correct responses, to have mistakes corrected, and to see the potential for improvement. Feedback should be given as soon as possible and summarized at a later time. It should be given in a positive manner, emphasizing what is correct. It should never include elements of ridicule or sarcasm, which would result in withdrawal from the learning situation. Feedback can be considered positive or negative in reference to established goals. Positive feedback would be the notation of goals achieved and negative feedback would be the goals that have yet to be

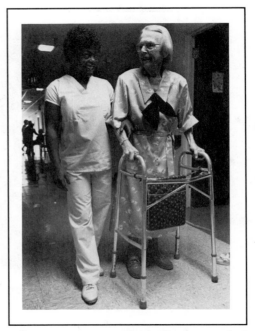

accomplished. Individual responses vary. Some persons prefer to focus on what they have accomplished, while others are mainly concerned with what is left to be accomplished.

Periodic Recall

Periodic recall of material facilitates retention for a longer period of time. Allowing time for recall at intervals is one reason that patient teaching should be started early in the hospitalization.

These principles are applicable to all learning. The same general ideas may be phrased in other ways. For example, motivation is a frequently listed principle. It is noted that a moderate degree of anxiety enhances learning. Also, the material must be meaningful to the learner. These are both facets of motivation. Another factor to consider is that learning requires energy and concentration. The patient must have enough energy available before any attempt at teaching is made.

CHECK IT OUT

With a small group of classmates analyze your instructor's approach to teaching. In the past three or four class sessions, how many teaching/learning principles have been applied? Some of these, such as active participation, should be your responsibility. Take into consideration that other factors such as repetitive practice of skills are not applicable to the normal classroom situation and that periodic recall should be evaluated over a semester. Remember that classroom teaching cannot be individualized.

Barriers to Learning

For the overall picture of learning, it is necessary to look at not only the factors that enhance learning but also any barriers or negative aspects. All of the principles discussed previously can be applied with no positive results if there is something standing in the way of learning. Barriers to learning include stress, sensory impairments, language, and barriers imposed by the nurse.

Stress

Excessive physical or emotional stress reduces the attention span and the capacity to learn. While some anxiety enhances learning, too much anxiety blocks learning. Emotional factors must be dealt with before intellectual factors can be approached. An extreme degree of anxiety causes the patient's attention to be focused on the cause of the anxiety and not on the new material. When under extreme stress, the patient and family may go through the motions of listening and answering at appropriate times, but little or no information is retained. Until the emotional stress is reduced, attempts to teach are futile.

Physiological stress can be as much a barrier as emotional stress. A seriously ill patient will not have the energy required to listen. The presence of pain will block input and make teaching ineffective. The physiological problem must be relieved before teaching can be effective.

Sensory Impairments

The patient may have visual or hearing impairments. These barriers can be overcome easily if the nurse is aware of them and plans the presentation accordingly. Visually impaired persons need large print and pictures to enhance learning. Persons with hearing impairments require more written material for future reference.

Language

There may be a language barrier present that makes the individual unable to learn. This may involve a foreign language or the use of terms the patient does not understand.

Barriers Imposed by the Nurse

The nurse may unintentionally impose barriers in several ways. Patient cues that indicate a need for learning may be ignored. The nurse may be aware of the learning need and have a teaching plan, but the time planned for teaching may not be a time when the patient is ready to learn. The material may be presented in such a hurried manner that little learning takes place. The teaching may have been delayed until the day of discharge, when the patient's thoughts are on going home. The nurse may talk down to the patient. This may occur with elderly patients when the nurse sees them as being in their second childhood and talks to them accordingly.

GENERAL PRINCIPLES OF TEACHING

Teaching provides the environment, materials, and conditions for learning to occur. The application of the principles of learning to the teaching process is an essential activity in teaching. However, there are other factors and approaches that make teaching more effective. Many of these are related to the learning principles but are considered from a different angle for teaching. The general principles of teaching are listed in Figure 5-2.

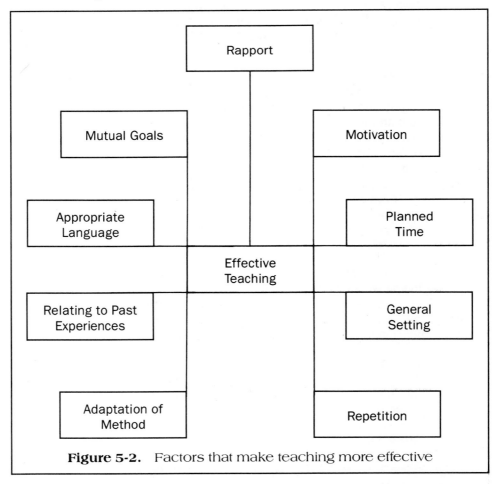

Figure 5-2.　Factors that make teaching more effective

Factors That Make Teaching More Effective

Teaching is a type of communication in which there are specific goals. Various activities are planned that relate to each goal. Teaching involves an interaction between teacher and learner in which both participants have an active role. Patient teaching is a process that follows the nursing process in format. There must be assessment, goal setting, planning, activities, and evaluation. The entire process revolves around helping the patient meet mutually acceptable goals. Factors that make teaching more effective include rapport, mutual goals, motivation, appropriate language, planned time, relating to past experiences, general setting, adaptation of method, and repetition.

Rapport

One of the first concerns in teaching is to establish rapport with the learner. Through communication, the nurse establishes a positive relationship and an atmosphere of caring and respect. This relationship not only makes the teaching more effective but also increases adherence on the part of the patient.

Mutual Goals

Goals must be mutually acceptable to both patient and nurse. Setting a goal can help the patient see the need for the information. A degree of bargaining may be necessary in establishing goals. For example, the nurse's goal may be to teach the patient to give self-injections of insulin. The patient may not like the idea of self-injection and may ask that a family member or members be taught the technique. This could be an acceptable solution to both patient and nurse if family members are agreeable and would be available whenever necessary to give the injections.

Motivation

The patient must be motivated to learn. There should be a desire to acquire the additional information and an awareness that the facts or skills are essential to the patient's present or future well-being. The patient must believe that the need will be met through the teaching/learning process. If a good relationship has been established between patient and nurse, the nurse may be able to motivate the patient by pointing out how the information will be useful. For example, the patient could be shown how a diet and exercise program can help prevent a future heart attack. Individuals who do not want to learn can be motivated when they see a need for the learning.

Appropriate Language

The use of understandable language is a high priority in patient teaching. Assessing the learner before preparing a teaching plan assures that the terminology will be understood. If a teaching plan that will be used for more than one patient is being prepared, the substitution of lay terms for medical terms is essential. Even with the use of lay terms, it may be necessary to make additional adjustments in the language or to use charts and diagrams to help an individual patient understand the material.

Planned Time

There must be a planned time and a comfortable environment for teaching to be effective. The time should be planned around hospital routines when there is the least likelihood of interruptions. Ample time must be allowed to present the material. If the nurse enters the room hurriedly and gives the patient a list of instructions that are only briefly reviewed, results will be negative.

Relating to Past Experiences

New knowledge and skills are most effectively taught when related to past experiences of the patient. Through assessment, the nurse determines areas in the patient's past to which the current teaching relates. For example, one patient had taught in a private nursery school and had applied numerous Band-Aids to children. When teaching this patient about a dressing change, the nurse related the procedure to the simple task of applying Band-Aids and added further information about sterile technique.

General Setting

Creating a physical environment conducive to learning is the same as that discussed for communication (see p. 51). Attention must be given to lighting, temperature, ventilation, privacy, noise, and pleasant surroundings. The psychological environment is in the hands of the nurse, who must create a nonjudgmental atmosphere in which the learner does not feel threatened. Any efforts made by the learner must be accepted. Errors should be corrected and praise given for correct responses. There should be no hint of criticism.

Adaptation of Method

In any presentation there must be an adaptation of the method to the content. Various methods seem to be equally effective, but each has characteristics that make it more valuable in specific situations. Skills should be demonstrated and ample time allowed for practice. Discussions regarding pathophysiology should be accompanied by diagrams. Activities should be planned that help the learner meet the accepted goals. If the activities are not effective, they should be replaced.

Repetition

Repetition of content increases the effectiveness of teaching. This may be done by presenting the same facts in a different manner or by summarizing important points at intervals. A summary in written form at the end of the teaching program gives the patient something concrete for reference after discharge.

These guidelines are suggestions for teaching that will increase the learner's understanding and retention of material presented. These general principles should be considered when presenting material in patient teaching.

Areas of Difficulty in Teaching

Any barrier to learning can hinder teaching. Careful assessment of the patient before presenting any information will avoid many of these barriers. However, there are other factors that make teaching difficult, such as the time factor, importance attached to teaching, lack of family involvement, and reaching goals.

The Time Factor

For busy health care workers the primary obstacle to patient teaching is lack of time. This is a legitimate concern. Additional responsibilities and a reduced staff often leave nurses without enough time to plan and carry out many of the activities they would like to include in patient care. However, the problem may involve more than a lack of time. The nurse may view patient education as an overwhelming task. It must be kept in mind that teaching can take place during routine care. The ability to communicate the knowledge and skill that the nurse possesses is all that is necessary to teach.

Importance Attached

Some nurses may believe that patient teaching is not important or that it should be the responsibility of the physician. These misconceptions can rob the patient of the information needed for care after discharge and/or the ability to maintain independence.

Lack of Family Involvement

Lack of family involvement can make teaching difficult. The patient usually needs a support person at home. The procedures may be too difficult for the patient to perform alone, the patient may need a period of time to regain strength to do the procedures, or there may be a memory problem. The nurse should make every effort to include a family member or a friend in patient education.

Failure to Reach Goals

Once teaching is begun, it must continue until the goals are met. The teaching effort should include all of the nursing team so that other members can reinforce the primary nurse's teaching plan. Personnel from other departments in the health care agency may be asked to help meet the goals if the patient's learning needs are in their field. A teaching effort discontinued in the middle may be worse than one never begun.

TEACHING STRATEGIES

Teaching strategies or methods are limited only by the instructor's imagination. Any of the methods can have numerous adaptations. Primary strategies are most commonly used in patient education. However, special strategies can be more effective in some situations. Each method must be adapted to the specific content and to the individual patient. Primary and special strategies can also be used in combination, as summarized in Figure 5-3.

Primary Strategies

Primary strategies in patient education include oral presentation, discussion, and demonstration.

Oral Presentation

The term "education" or "teaching" usually calls to mind the image of a classroom with a teacher at the front of the class. This concept would usually be termed a lecture. In one-to-one situations oral presentation may be a preferable label because it has a less formal classroom connotation. It is an efficient method of imparting information to a number of people, but it is not the most effective strategy in many situations. There is little room for interaction in this type of presentation, and it can be boring for the learner if it is very long. To be most effective, oral presentations should incorporate other methods or aids.

Discussion

Discussion is an effective strategy in patient education. It requires learner participation with active interchange between the learner and teacher. It can be used as a means of assessing the individual's knowledge while giving the necessary information to the patient. Discussion is especially useful in group teaching. Learners exchange ideas among themselves and often are more comfortable knowing that others have and are willing to talk about problems similar to their own.

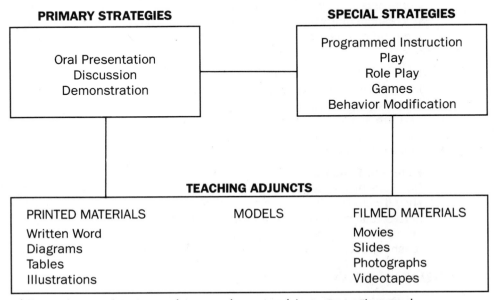

Figure 5-3.   Primary and secondary teaching strategies and teaching adjuncts.

Demonstration

Demonstration by the nurse with a return demonstration by the patient is the strategy of choice for psychomotor skills. It encompasses the cognitive and psychomotor domains of learning and involves visual, auditory, and kinesthetic modes of learning. The patient watches the demonstration, then performs the procedure. The rationale for each step is stressed during the demonstration. This method should be presented in individual or small group situations because it is difficult for the patient to see details of the procedure in a large group.

Practice time must be allowed following the demonstration. Some practice can be unsupervised, but the nurse must check frequently to ensure that proper techniques are being used. Patients may be nervous in return demonstrations, so private sessions for evaluating performance of a procedure are often preferable.

Special Strategies

Special teaching strategies may at times be more effective than primary ones. Some special strategies are useful in specific situations, while others require more time than is available. All of these strategies require careful patient assessment to determine the probable patient response. Special teaching strategies include programmed instruction, play, role play, games, and behavior modification.

Programmed Instruction

Some patients can benefit from the use of programmed instruction. This is a form of learning in which a small amount of material is presented followed by questions. The selection of an answer includes directions either to proceed to the next question if the right answer was chosen or to review the question if the wrong answer was chosen. Sometimes the answer is concealed until the student has had an opportunity to answer the question, when it can be checked. Many programs of this type are available on computers. This is a type of active learner participation. It can be individually paced; however, some individuals find it boring and will not use it to advantage. The learner must be literate and self-motivated. There is little teacher/learner interaction with programmed instruction. If this type of instruction is to accomplish the intended purpose, the nurse must devise a means of evaluating the patient's knowledge during and at the completion of the program.

Play

Play is a teaching strategy that is very effective with children. It helps to stimulate cognitive processes and organize the child's thinking. However, the child's physical condition must be considered, since play requires energy. Very sick children would not be able to participate.

Role Play

In role play each participant is assigned to or selects a role and the dialogue is ad-libbed with no prior rehearsal. This approach is effective in helping patients understand chronic conditions such as diabetes. It can give patients insights into handling home health care situations. It is somewhat time-consuming. The participants must be willing to put themselves into the situation. It keeps the learner involved at all times and shows how problems might be dealt with by others.

Games

Games can be useful with many age groups if the participants are interested in this approach. Competition is involved, which makes it especially applicable to the school-age child. Adults may or may not like competition or games in general, and some might have difficulty in following directions and applying the ideas presented. This is a nonthreatening activity that involves the participants and allows patients to apply previously learned facts. It, too, is time-consuming.

Behavior Modification

Behavior modification techniques have been tried in some situations. This is based on the premise that a person's behaviors are under conscious control and can be strengthened, eliminated, or replaced. This approach rewards desirable behavior and ignores undesirable actions. There is no type of criticism or punishment involved. Sometimes learning contracts are combined with behavior modification; for example, a reward or bonus is earned when a task is completed by the patient.

Behavior modification can have positive results but must be continued over a period of time. It is not generally applicable to short-term hospitalization.

Adjuncts to Teaching (Teaching Aids)

Teaching adjuncts, or teaching aids, include any audiovisual materials that can be used to enhance the teaching process, such as printed materials, models, and filmed materials. They are not intended to be used as a primary method of teaching but as accompaniments to make teaching more effective.

Printed Materials

Printed materials are useful adjuncts to other methods but are not effective without nurse-patient interaction. The written word gives visual reinforcement to oral instructions and serves as a source for future reference. Diagrams and tables can be used to show relationships. Simple diagrams are excellent for use with children. Anatomical illustrations can be useful with any group to help explain pathophysiology.

Models

The use of models may be more effective than diagrams. However, they are expensive, and the average health care facility will not have an unlimited number available. Models encourage learner participation as patients manipulate them.

Filmed Materials

Films can impart information in a way that is readily remembered. Films may be especially helpful to patients with limited reading skills. They may not be effective for elderly persons since patients cannot proceed at their own pace, as they can with printed material. Films take time to set up and involve some expense, but they may be an excellent aid for use in affective teaching, especially if followed by group discussion. Films should only be used in conjunction with discussion.

Slide presentations are often used in a similar way, but the lack of motion does not make them as realistic. Photographs can be used to show actual patient situations.

Videotapes have become increasingly popular. The equipment is much simpler to set up and the tapes provide the same advantages and limitations as films. Some health care facilities are using closed-circuit television to present tapes on selected conditions at specific times during the day so that patients and families can view the films in their rooms.

All prepared teaching aids must be reviewed before being used because they may not contain the information desired or needed by the patient. Any printed, illustrated, or filmed presentation or model must be considered supplemental and not the only method of delivering information to the patient. These are best preceded and/or followed by individual or group nurse-patient contact for the information to be meaningful.

CHECK IT OUT

Select one favorite teacher and one of the least liked teachers.

Make a list for each with the following information.
1. Teaching strategy used most of time.
2. Special teaching strategies used at intervals.
3. How often various adjuncts to teaching are used.

Compare the two lists. How much of an impact did the strategies and adjuncts have on your enjoyment of the course?

Some basic considerations in the teaching/learning process have been presented. They are suggestions that can be applied to make patient teaching more effective. As students become experienced in patient teaching, they will develop techniques that are comfortable for them and are well received by patients.

◖ IN A CAPSULE ◗

The *basic domains of learning* involve cognitive, affective, and psychomotor aspects. *Learning modes* are individual preferences for an approach to learning; people may be global or linear learners; they may prefer visual, auditory, or kinesthetic activities. *Factors that enhance learning* include diverse aspects such as consideration of learner's rate and mode of learning, intellectual capacity, meaningful material, satisfaction, realistic goals, degree of anxiety, successful efforts, proceeding from simple to complex, use of several senses, active participation, repetitive practice, application, positive feedback, and periodic recall. Excess stress can be a *barrier to learning*, as can hearing or visual impairments and language usage.

Factors that make teaching more effective include rapport, mutual goals, motivation, appropriate language, planned time, relating to past experiences, general setting, adaptation of method, and repetition. *Teaching may be hindered* by the time factor, importance attached to teaching, lack of family involvement, and failure to continue until goals are met.

The *primary teaching strategies* that nurses utilize are lecture or oral presentation, discussion, and demonstration. *Special strategies* that are very effective in many situations include programmed instruction, play, role play, games, and behavior modification. *Adjuncts to teaching* (teaching aids) include models and printed or filmed material, which serve as an aid in teaching but should not be used in place of teacher/learner contact.

DO YOU REMEMBER

- the basic domains of learning?
- several modes of learning?
- primary barriers to learning?
- items that may hinder teaching?
- the three primary patient teaching strategies?

CAN YOU DESCRIBE

- factors tht enhance learning?
- factors to be considered that increase the effectiveness of teaching?
- the application of special strategies in teaching?
- the use of adjuncts to teaching strategies?

ACTION, PLEASE

1. You are working as an RN on a medical unit. One of your assigned patients is Mr. Hamilton, a 54-year-old owner of a small successful business. He works long hours managing the business and experiences the usual stresses. He has recently developed high blood pressure. You are showing him a videotape on hypertension.

a. Give circumstances under which each of the following options might be used.

b. Give the rationale for using each option.

c. Note the applicable teaching/learning principle for each.

1. Leave a booklet on hypertension with him.

　a. _____

　b. _____

　c. _____

2. Review the videotape the next day with him.

　a. _____

　b. _____

　c. _____

3. Discuss the information presented immediately.

　a. _____

　b. _____

　c. _____

4. Use questions and answers to evaluate the effectiveness.

　a. _____

　b. _____

　c. _____

Which option or combination do you consider most effective for Mr. Hamilton?

2. *Application of Principles.* You are formulating a teaching plan to instruct a 32-year-old man about dressing changes following an injury to his lower leg. How would you apply the following teaching/learning principles?

a. Realistic goal setting is essential to learning.

_____

_____

_____

b. The patient must be motivated to learn.

_____

_____

_____

c. Learning is increased when more than one of the senses is involved.

_____

_____

_____

d. Success in learning breeds success.

_____

_____

_____

e. Repetitive practice is essential for learning skills.

_____

_____

_____

6

The Nurse Promotes Patient Education in the Health Care Setting

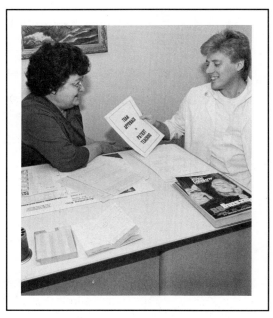

OBJECTIVES

Upon completion of this chapter, the student will be able to:

- list the general purposes of patient teaching.
- discuss positive and negative factors in patient adherence to the prescribed regimen.
- describe areas in which the nurse promotes patient independence.
- list general basic information needs of patients.
- describe the role of communication in helping the patient learn to cope.
- discuss the legal responsibility of the nurse in patient education.
- note the circumstances under which registered nurses can delegate teaching responsibilities.
- relate patient advocacy to patient education.
- state the manner in which health professionals prove the effectiveness of patient teaching.
- describe the process of making

Put your feet in the right place, and then stand firm.
Abraham Lincoln

changes in a patient education program.
- state approaches of the nurse that tend to increase physicians' cooperation in patient education.
- note advantages of interdisciplinary planning for patient education programs.

GLOSSARY OF TERMS*

Adherence   Observance of routine by choice.
Bargaining   A positive process through which both parties derive satisfaction.
Coercion   Enforcement by threats; cause to do by pressure.
Confrontation   To bring opposing ideas face-to-face.
Cope   Deal with and attempt to overcome problems and difficulties.

*Definitions applicable to content.

Education is one of the patient's rights. It is also an important function and legal obligation of the nurse. The overall goal of patient education is to inform patients and their families about the current illness, related diagnostic and treatment modalities, and other pertinent health-related information. The results of the teaching, hopefully, will be adherence to the recommended regimen and behavioral changes necessary to maintain health.

GENERAL PURPOSES OF PATIENT TEACHING

The nurse's approach to patient education must be more than to simply meet legal obligations or avoid lawsuits. The goal of patient education is to help the patient maintain as high a quality of life as possible. The purposes of patient teaching are summarized in Figure 6.1 and discussed in the following pages.

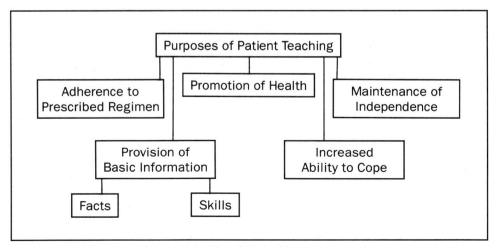

Figure 6.1   Teaching with a purpose

Promotion of Health

Through effective teaching, nurses can help people maintain optimum health. This should be the aim of members of all health professions. While physical care is the most visible component, the maintenance of health is a goal that all health care providers strive to accomplish. However, sometimes this goal is not met. Nurses attempt to teach hospitalized patients methods of preventing recurrences of the present pathological condition as well as prevention of other illnesses. However, sometimes patients do not take advantage of this information.

General hygienic measures are routinely reviewed with patients. Preventive medicine is promoted by all health practitioners as well as by many public agencies. Effective patient education can increase positive responses to preventive health programs. Nurses should take the lead in emphasizing promotion of health. This should be one aspect of patient teaching during hospitalization.

Adherence to Prescribed Regimen

A problem frequently encountered in medical treatment is patients' lack of adherence to a prescribed regimen after discharge. Compliance is a term frequently used to refer to maintaining the prescribed regimen. Adherence seems to be a better term, however, since compliance has the connotation of yielding to another's will. Adherence implies free will in following a set of instructions. Patients need to feel that they have a choice in and a certain amount of control over what happens to them. Members of the health care team too often tend to assume an authority position with subtle threats to withdraw support if directions are not followed. They sometimes place the nurse/patient relationship in a parent/child position.

The relationship of the patient and health care provider is a two-way street. The patient expects a high degree of accountability on the part of the health professionals. The health care team expects the patient to take the responsibility for adherence, and more emphasis should be placed on this.

Forms of Nonadherence

Nonadherence can be seen in various forms, all of which can have serious effects. Medications may not be taken at all or may not be taken in the prescribed manner. Too much or too little medication may be taken, or it may not be taken at recommended times or in relation to meals. Side-effects that the patient has been instructed to report may be ignored. Doctors' appointments may not be kept.

Recommendations in the areas of diet and life-style changes are frequently ignored. For example, Mr. Peterson's physician prescribed a low-cholesterol diet and daily exercise after a mild heart attack. Mr. Peterson followed the regimen for 2 weeks before he returned to his sedentary routines and diet including many fried foods.

Even instructions for mild forms of treatment such as hot or cold applications, dressings, or supports may be ignored. Suggestions for inoculations for disease prevention may not be considered important and may soon be forgotten.

Reasons for Nonadherence

The nursing profession is aware of the problem of nonadherence. Noncompliance is an accepted nursing diagnosis. This is partly related to knowledge deficit, since increased knowledge may be associated with increased adherence. But patient education is not the only answer. There is no clear-cut answer to this problem. Effective patient education seems to be a factor, since people cannot be expected to follow instructions they do not understand. The average person will not become involved in following a rigorous routine if not made aware of the value of the program. Other factors such as age, socioeconomic status, and seriousness of illness have been considered but have not been shown to be definite factors in adherence.

Psychosocial Factors in Adherence

Some psychosocial influences seem to be related to adherence. The person who values health tends to accept the recommended regimen in order to return to good health. For example, Mrs. Butler has numerous allergies but avoids contact with those things that trigger reactions because she wants to be able to care for her three school-age children. People who tend to use illness as a means of escaping responsibility and gaining attention make little effort to change patterns that would improve health status. Mrs. Packman is also plagued by allergies. She has discovered that her allergic reactions gain attention for her from her husband. She sometimes consciously comes in contact with offending substances and delays taking medication in order to get extra attention.

Nonadherence may be related to a denial of the illness or a view of illness as a sign of weakness. In a preceding example, Mr. Peterson, who had a heart attack, decided that his heart was fine and that there was no need for him to follow his doctor's orders.

Routines recommended by the physician may interfere with a person's life-style or job. The person may have a lack of faith in medications in general or may have had an adverse reaction to medication in the past that resulted in distrust of all medications. Finances can hinder adherence if expensive drugs and appliances are recommended. Reasons for nonadherence are often difficult to pinpoint and may be even more difficult to overcome.

Adherence is a complex entity with many emotional overtones. A high or low anxiety level seems to be a factor in nonadherence, while an average or normal level of anxiety contributes to adherence. The patient must be motivated to carry out the procedures prescribed and follow the recommended routines. The nurse must establish a positive relationship through communication to motivate the patient and secure cooperation. Through this positive relationship, the nurse is able to provide more effective patient teaching and hopefully enhance adherence.

Maintenance of Independence

A primary goal of nurses in patient education is to assist patients to return to their former level of functioning. This is related to adherence because many patients do not receive maximum benefit from medical treatment because of nonadherence to recommendations after discharge. Patients may face an enormous task in attempting to comply with therapeutic regimens. If, for example, the equipment is complicated, the routine is time-consuming, or the regimen is distasteful to the patient, it may not be followed.

Patient teaching can be a factor in helping the patient adhere to the prescribed regimen. For example, Mrs. Jackson seldom practiced breathing exercises for emphysema until the nurse used diagrams to explain the pathophysiology of emphysema and the benefits to be gained from the routine. If persons do not understand why carrying out certain procedures will benefit them, the chance of adherence is slim. Education does not assure adherence, but it is a means of motivating the patient's efforts.

The goal or purpose of the nurse may be to help the patient learn to function when there are physical impairments. These may have resulted from an accident or a major illness. The nurse can be a prime influence in supporting the patient and family in learning to use prostheses, in accepting a limitation in activities, or in adjusting routines to provide the physical care necessary. Patient teaching may be one of the most important functions of the nurse in caring for patients who have conditions that require readjustment of activities of daily living. The teaching frequently extends well beyond the period of hospitalization if many changes must be made. Emotional support given by the nurse is often as important as teaching psychomotor skills. The more patients are able to accept physical handicaps, the more independently they will be able to live.

CHECK IT OUT

Work with a small group of students. Select a patient whose level of functioning is descreased as a result of a recent accident or physical dysfunction. The patient should be familiar to at least one member of the group.
1. List the areas in which the patient is now dependent on others, for example, mobility, eating, bathing, dressing, etc.
2. Note specific aids that would enable the patient to function more independently in each of the areas noted.
3. Determine approaches the nurse could use to encourage independence.

Provision of Basic Information

Patient education deals with supplying information in any areas that will enable the patient to maintain or improve health status. The need for information may be expressed either by the patient or by the nurse. Learning needs should be a part of all patient care plans. In fact a patient care plan may not be considered complete without a nursing diagnosis denoting a learning need. Patient education is one of the functions of the nurse. It is an integral part of comprehensive patient care. The patient's learning needs must be met to enable the patient to maintain a high level of functioning. The information should be presented to the patient in a manner in which the patient can most effectively cope with the current illness and function at a high level in the future.

Facts

Factual information about the hospital routines is usually the first step in patient education. Hospital orientation is carried out shortly after a patient is admitted. Orientation may not be considered in the true realm of patient teaching, but it can make a difference in the patient's satisfaction and adherence during the hospital stay. The patient should never have to ask to find out how to call a nurse when needed, what time meals are expected, the times of visiting hours, or any of the hospital routines.

Factual information about the disease process for which the patient was admitted may be an information need of the patient. There is usually a degree of anxiety if the patient is not familiar with the diagnosis. An explanation to the patient in understandable terms of the pathophysiological changes that occur in the body during a particular disease process helps the patient to accept what is going on. For example, Mrs. Curry was very concerned about symptoms of a potassium deficit resulting from medications. Her anxiety was relieved when the nurse explained the occurrence and means of reversing the imbalance. Giving information promotes the nurse-patient relationship. The patient sees the nurse as someone who is knowledgeable as well as empathic by being caring enough to take time to give full explanations.

The information needed might be specifics of a dietary regimen. It is not sufficient to hand a patient a diet list of foods that can be eaten and others that must be avoided. Explanations of the reasons for certain items being included or excluded are essential if the patient is to adhere to the diet.

Any measures that enhance the full recovery or promote the general health of the patient should be included in patient education. The patient may need information about general hygienic practices. Nurses may assume that everyone is knowledgeable regarding hygiene but this is not always true. Nurses care for patients from all walks of life and every socioeconomic status. Knowledge cannot be assumed because of the age or economic status of the patient. The nurse must assess each patient individually to determine need for information about basic hygiene practices.

Important information needed by patients is that concerned with medications. Too often medications are not taken properly because the patient does not understand the reasons for taking the medicine as prescribed. Careful explanations of reasons for taking a medication at a certain time, taking it with or without food, the effects of the medication in the body, the dangers of omitting or changing dosages, and possible side-effects will enhance the willingness of the patient to follow directions. The patient should be made aware of side-effects that should be reported to the physician. Any explanations that are given must be in terms that are understandable to the patient and should be repeated or written as necessary.

Skills

Some skills are necessary for long periods of time for ongoing maintenance of health. Insulin injections, colostomy irrigations, or tube feedings may be skills that the patient and/or family will need for maintaining life as well as health. These procedures may need to be continued for the remainder of the patient's life. The rationale for the procedures must be stressed so that the routine will be closely followed. The teaching should take place well before discharge so that sufficient supervised practice time is available.

The patient may need skills for short-term usage to recover from a current illness. Dressing changes, wound irrigations, and special skin care may be for only a short period but are necessary for recovery. The patient or family may need to change the dressings for just a few days or weeks, but inability to perform the procedure correctly may lead to an infection that will necessitate readmission to the hospital. The patient's or family's ability to follow directions must be carefully evaluated to assure that the teaching was effective and/or that the procedure was performed correctly.

Some skills deal with restoration of function. Nurses must often teach the patient exercises for regaining muscle strength, for example, after an accident. New skills may be necessary for performing activities of daily living. After a stroke, for example, the patient must learn to make adaptations in simple tasks such as eating that may require the use of special utensils. Part of the patient teaching program may include allowing the patient to become familiar with special equipment during hospitalization. This may take place in a rehabilitation center. Patient education is not reserved for hospitalized patients. It includes all health care settings.

Increased Ability to Cope

One of the most difficult tasks of the nurse may be helping the patient learn to cope with a permanent disability or a devastating prognosis. Coping involves facing problems and difficulties and attempting to overcome them. Coping is a part of everyday life in dealing with minor problems that arise, but patients' problems and difficulties are usually more complex. The patient may need to learn to cope with a chronic health problem or a terminal illness. Helping the patient meet this need is a facet of patient education.

The patient may need to learn to cope with a decreased level of functioning or a major adjustment in life-style. In this case the teaching will include factual and skill components, but the application of effective communication skills will be one of the most important aspects. The nurse can help the patient cope by listening and by giving emotional support. The patient must accept an illness and learn to cope with limitations for any degree of quality of life to be maintained. Problems must be brought out in the open and verbalized so that they can be dealt with in a way that enables the patient to accept the situation. Because coping is a first step, the nurse can promote verbalization of concerns and support the patient emotionally to look at and accept the facts. Communication skills are intertwined with teaching skills to provide maximum benefit to the patient.

RESPONSIBILITY FOR PATIENT EDUCATION

Patient/family education is considered a function of the nurse and other health professionals, but this function is not always effectively fulfilled. Nursing organizations, nursing theorists and clinicians, hospital associations, and hospital accreditation agencies all stress the need for quality patient education. Patients consistently express a need for more comprehensive information about their illness and care.

Legal Responsibility of the Nurse

Nurses have a legal responsibility for patient education. Most state Nurse Practice Acts list this as a function of the nurse. For the few that do not, their laws may be displaced by the patient's right to know. If the knowledge is critical to the patient's health, patient teaching will be viewed as a legal responsibility of the nurse. Students as well as practicing professional nurses are included in this category, because patients have the right to expect competent nursing care at all times when hospitalized.

Local standards are a consideration in deciding legal responsibility. Job descriptions of nursing positions usually include patient teaching. Hospitals establish standards for continuity of care. This includes patient education if the care is to be truly comprehensive. Even though it is not as visible as physical care, patient teaching is essential. Patients must know how to adequately care for themselves after discharge.

The registered nurse may choose to delegate a portion of the teaching responsibilities to other knowledgeable nurses but remains responsible for what is delegated. The results of patient teaching are the responsibility and within the scope of practice of the RN. This is particularly true when the RN delegates responsibilities to a licensed practical nurse. For example, if an RN prepares a patient for a series of gastrointestinal studies, the LPN who is assigned to care for the patient can reinforce the teaching and more specifically explain the procedure to the patient. In evaluating the effectiveness of the teaching, the RN would consider how the LPN had been prepared and supervised in this situation.

Patient Advocacy Related to Patient Teaching

If nurses are to assume the role of patient advocate, the assurance that the patient receives the essential information for care is part of this role. If nurses do not monitor patient teaching, other organizations may take the role of patient advocate. They will demand better nursing care and fulfillment of the patient's right to obtain complete information regarding the diagnosis and treatment while hospitalized. Patients are aware of the necessity of adequate information regarding their illness and care. Patients commonly complain that no one will take the time to explain things to them. They may complain that readmission to a hospital stemmed from lack of information regarding care after discharge.

Accountability for Patient Education

Establishment of quality patient care standards, including patient education, is encouraged by professional associations. The general public demands quality health care. Standards of care are used in self-evaluation and peer review to maintain accountability of nurses in verifying provision of quality care to patients. The established standards are a guideline, but the actual implementation is the factor that must be observed.

Health professionals must be able to prove the effectiveness of patient teaching efforts. Documentation provides the evidence that adequate patient/family teaching was a part of the comprehensive care provided. Careful documentation of patient/family teaching should note the response of the patient and/or family to the material presented. Nurses and health care agencies have avoided lawsuits or been able to win cases in which the documentation clearly showed the extent of the teaching, the patient's or family's ability to perform procedures, or that the instructions given were understood.

PROMOTION OF PATIENT EDUCATION PROGRAMS

The quality of patient education may leave something to be desired. Even though it is one of the rights of the patient, it is part of nurses' job descriptions, it is considered a legal responsibility of the nurse and other health professionals, and it is documented as having been accomplished, the end results are not always what they could or should be.

There must be cooperation of the nursing team for patient education to be effective. Communication among the members of the nursing team is basic. One nurse may plan and start teaching a patient, but other nurses need to continue and/or reinforce the teaching in order for it to be effective.

The nurse can be important in establishing a more effective program of patient education in the health care setting. Support of other departments in the facility is essential to put a program into effect, but peer commitment is a key factor in the actual application of any patient education program. Figure 6-2 illustrates what can be accomplished by a staff nurse who sees a need in patient education and is willing to work toward meeting that need.

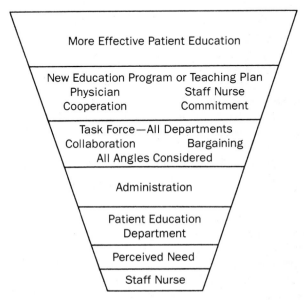

More Effective Patient Education

New Education Program or Teaching Plan
Physician   Staff Nurse
Cooperation   Commitment

Task Force—All Departments
Collaboration   Bargaining
All Angles Considered

Administration

Patient Education
Department

Perceived Need

Staff Nurse

Figure 6.2   An idea grows and the patient wins

Collaboration in Establishing a Program

Patient education cannot be successfully accomplished by a single nurse working with one patient. It is true that students are taught to develop teaching plans for an individual patient covering a single aspect of care. This is a learning situation for the student and not meant to cover all of the learning needs of that patient. The entire nursing team must be involved to establish any kind of continuity in the teaching/learning process. For a program of patient education in a health care agency to be successful, there must be cooperation among all departments as well as the nursing team members.

Securing Approval for Change

Most health care institutions have some form of patient education standards. The implementation of these standards may or may not adequately meet learning needs of patients. Various approaches may be used in different areas of the hospital. Some may be more effective than others. The nurse who is aware of deficiencies in the patient education program and has some ideas regarding new or better approaches can work toward putting these ideas into action. Any changes that may be brought about must take place within the general organizational framework of the institution. The nurse must know the hierarchical structure and proper channels through which to work.

The department responsible for patient education must be the one that initiates any change in this direction. The idea may simply be presented to the responsible department, or the nurse may want to be involved in the mechanics of making any changes. If the nurse is qualified to work toward putting a change into effect in the patient education program, it will be necessary to secure the cooperation of the administration. Any new programs or changes will be time-consuming and involve expense to the hospital. But that does not alter the fact that a staff nurse can be instrumental in creating a new program or new approach to patient education if willing to invest the time and effort necessary.

Before presenting ideas to the proper department or committee, the nurse should determine currently available printed or filmed resource materials. Most health care agencies have materials on hand. The hospital library and nursing stations should be checked for materials. Educational services personnel or committee members can be asked for assistance in locating pertinent materials. Outside sources of free or low-cost materials include pharmaceutical and medical supply companies, the state health department, and the Government Printing Office in Washington, D.C. A list of resources available and additional material sources will indicate the nurse's dedication to improving the patient education program and should increase chances of obtaining approval.

Organizing a Task Force

If approval is obtained for planning a change in the patient education program, a task force is usually formed and given the responsibility for proposing a detailed plan. The task force must work within the policies of the health care agency and accept decisions of the administration. The nurse or other person who is the chairman or collaborator in setting up the program must try to obtain support of all departments. By enlisting personnel from all departments and seeking their input, a spirit of mutual cooperation and appreciation is established. Even though the person serving as chairman for the task force may have very definite ideas of the direction to proceed, requesting and objectively considering ideas of the others will increase cooperation.

Recognition of the others on the task force as experts and acknowledging their contributions and capabilities creates an atmosphere in which the patient will eventually benefit. High-quality patient education will then become a reality. By not asserting the power or authority of the chairman, decision making is usually facilitated. Each member must be willing to share expertise, thus preventing negative reactions related to felt ownership of patients. When contributions of all members are recognized, the task force enjoys a pleasant working relationship as well as the respect of others for their accomplishments.

Working Within the Task Force

In working with a group in making changes in the patient education program, various tactics are employed. To realize maximum results within the group, there must be some bargaining. This can best be accomplished in a rational and calm atmosphere with any emotional responses ignored. An agreeable bargain might be reached where the goals for a patient education program remain the same but the content and methods undergo some change. Negotiating a bargain is a give-and-take affair. Both parties must be willing to give in some areas. Effective use of bargaining avoids confrontation.

Direct confrontation usually produces an emotional response. The term itself has negative overtones. This method should never be used to force ideas on another person but may be a method to encourage a new approach to a problem. In confrontation, opposing ideas are presented. Ideally, these proposals are discussed by the entire group with the strengths and weaknesses of each discussed. This approach can be used to clarify the perceptions of each member and to compare the positive and negative aspects of the different viewpoints.

Coercion is strictly a last-ditch effort. It forces people to do things against their will. Pointing out the legal responsibilities in patient education as a means to implement the program can be considered coercion. While it may force the members to cooperate, it is not the most desirable means to the end. The participants will not enter wholeheartedly into the implementation of the plan and the results may be less effective than anticipated.

Considering the proposal from a different angle can be effective. When patient education is viewed in the light of an attempt to gain patient adherence, it can be considered similar to informed consent. The information can be given to the patient, who is then responsible for making a decision. This introduces a different perspective and may gain the cooperation of some who had been opposed to the proposed program.

Implementing a Change

While planning for the future, the present must be considered. Any plans for a patient education program must be realistic in all contexts. Will the nurses have time to implement the program? Will all departments cooperate? Will the program provide effective education for all patients? Are all essentials for patient education covered? The proposed program may be put into effect in a small area and the results documented. The results may convince all concerned that the idea is an acceptable one. Regardless of difficulties encountered when attempting a change, the situation should be viewed in a positive light. If the physician wants teaching carried out only when specifically ordered, this should be considered as contributing to team effort rather than restricting activities of other health care personnel.

CHECK IT OUT

Determine the manner in which patient education is approached in your clinical facility.

> Is it included in the care plans?
> Are standardized patient teaching plans available?
> Are standardized plans individualized?
> Does patient teaching require a doctor's order?
> How much time do nurses devote to patient teaching?
> How well is patient teaching documented?
> How much informal teaching have you observed?

Compare your findings with those of students in other clinical facilities. Try to determine areas that need improvement.

Cooperation of Physicians in Patient Education Programs

All members of the health team should be involved in organizing the patient education program. However, it is the physician who deals most closely with the patient over a period of time. The physician's role is often a long-term relationship with the patient, sometimes having cared for the patient and possibly the patient's family for many years. Nurses and other health professionals see the patient for only a short period during hospitalization. Even though nurses tend to develop close ties in working with the patient on a daily basis, the nurse does not usually follow up on the patient after discharge. Both the doctor and the nurse tend to think in terms of "my patient," but this concept is one that can be detrimental to the patient. A better concept is for each to think in terms of "our patient." This can come about only through the use of effective communication in building good working relationships between physicians and nurses.

The physician is legally responsible for the overall care of the patient. Each physician has definite ideas about patient education. While the nurse has a legal responsibility for patient education, it must be conducted within the realm of authority of the physician. Nurses have functions independent of the physician, but other functions are in the category of carrying out the physician's orders. Many physicians are conscientious regarding patient education and take time to provide their patients with information necessary for understanding and self-care. When the physician prefers to do the patient teaching, the nurse should not assume that it will not be effectively carried out.

Areas of Misunderstanding

Some physicians may feel threatened by new roles the nurse is assuming. They see the nurse as a threat to their practice rather than a collaborator in efforts directed toward the good of the patient. The term "education" may convey a picture of an overly standardized classroom situation in which the same information is given to all. Patient education may be seen by the physician in terms of involved pathological explanations. Nurses must help the physician understand instructional approaches used by the nursing team. They must convey the idea that they are not attempting to take over the physician's role but to strengthen it.

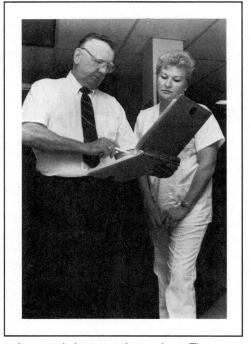

Physicians who resist patient education by nurses may have some concerns regarding the ability of nurses to teach their patients. They may fear that nurses do not have the knowledge base to adequately instruct the patient. They may see the nurses' teaching as superficial and not information the patient needs to know. On the other hand, the physician may not be aware of the learning needs of the patient. Sometimes physicians will give an explanation to the patient in terms that are not understood by the patient. The patient is hesitant to ask for a further explanation for fear of taking too much of the physician's time. Nurses frequently clarify the physician's explanations or instructions. Only by working together can patient needs be met.

The doctor may react to an aggressive approach on the part of the nurse. Some nurses attempt to invade the established role of the physician. Fortunately only a very small minority of nurses tend to put personal goals above the best interests of the patient. Most nurses want to work cooperatively with the doctor in providing quality care for the patient. Communication skills must be exercised in interactions with physicians as well as with patients. More can be accomplished with an attitude of cooperation than competitiveness.

Some physicians may believe that allowing the nurse to assume the role of patient educator will increase the possibility of a lawsuit. However, the opposite is actually true. Adequate information given to the patient will reduce the risk of malpractice suits. It will also lessen the number of telephone calls to the doctor caused by lack of information. If the doctor and nurse work together in patient education, the patient is the ultimate winner. There is better rapport between patient and physician when the patient understands the illness and the reasons for the treatment modality.

Promoting Cooperation of Physicians

One way in which the nurse can secure cooperation from the physician is to provide a written summary of points included in patient teaching and questions that the patient asked. This reflects the learning needs of the patient and gives specific points emphasized by the nurse. The nurse may not have been able to answer all of the questions adequately. These could be noted and the physician asked to clarify them.

Sometimes there may be a problem related to the terminology used. If there seems to be resistance to the term patient education, the terms patient teaching, patient instruction, or patient information could be used. Instead of using the term nurses' discharge summary, discharge information could be used. The results are the same regardless of the name given to the activity or to the form. The problem may not be in the terminology but in the manner in which it is presented to the physician. The physician should be informed of what is included in a patient teaching plan so that information can be added or deleted. The doctor should be made aware of the learning needs of patients. The nurse must put communication skills to work to secure cooperation.

It is essential to have the cooperation of physicians in order to have an effective patient education program. Input by physicians into the overall teaching program will help to assure their cooperation and add valuable material to each area of the program. Physicians can be one of the most valuable resources available to nurses in patient teaching.

Interdisciplinary Involvement in Patient Education

While it is important to have the cooperation of physicians in planning a program of patient education, other health professionals should not be overlooked. Members of each discipline within the health care organization have expertise that is part of the total care of the patient. The specialized knowledge of each can be invaluable in patient teaching. Figure 6-3 depicts the importance of departments working together to cover all aspects of patient education.

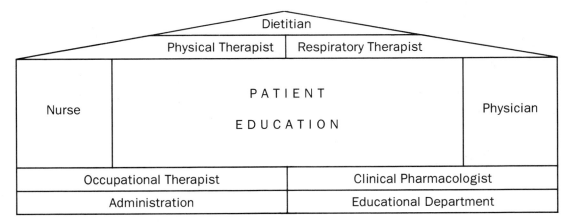

Figure 6.3 The house of patient education needs interdisciplinary coverage.

Pharmacologist

The vast majority of patients who are hospitalized will be given medications while in the hospital. Many will have to continue taking some medicines after discharge. The pharmacist is the logical health professional to give them the information needed. Some agencies have clinical pharmacologists who follow the progress of patients on various medications during their hospital stay. Their patient teaching can be a valuable asset to the overall education program. When a clinical pharmacologist is not available, the nurse can check with the pharmacist about any medication and relay the information to the patient.

Dietitian

Dietitians are an integral part of a comprehensive teaching program. Their functions include individualized planning of diets, communicating with patients regarding special requests, preparing diet instruction lists, and instructing patients regarding selection of foods on special diets. The dietitian should have a role in the planning as well as implementations of a patient teaching program.

Respiratory Therapist

Respiratory therapists should be included in the overall program planning and implementation. The therapist should explain any procedures and the expected results. Patients frequently must continue to use various pieces of respiratory equipment after discharge. While the nurse is familiar with much of the equipment, the respiratory therapist is better prepared to instruct the patient in the use, care, and precautions involved.

Physical and Occupational Therapists

The physical therapy and occupational therapy departments are equally important in patient education. Their roles are of prime importance in patient rehabilitation programs following strokes, accidents, or any condition requiring adaptation to different methods of performing daily activities. Members of these departments should be included in the planning phase as well as the implementation of patient education programs.

It might seem that such an array of teachers would overwhelm the patient. However, the patient more likely feels secure in knowing that each person involved in teaching is an expert in that field. In college, students want instructors who are knowledgeable in their field. This is somewhat the same approach.

The program should be planned so that the teaching is carried out a little at a time. Patient teaching as well as discharge planning should begin when the patient is admitted to the hospital.

Patient education is a part of comprehensive patient care. Immediate aspects of physical care often take attention away from it. However, patient education cannot be overlooked if total patient care is the concern of the nurse. Adequate patient teaching often prevents needless rehospitalization for the same condition. Patient teaching is slanted toward the health end of the health-illness continuum. The goal of all health professionals should be optimum health and level of functioning for patients under their care. Effective patient education contributes to this.

Insights into the problems and possibilities in planning a patient education program give a better understanding of the overall picture, even though many nurses will never be involved in initiating a new program. Nurses are legally responsible for effective patient education. For a program to be most beneficial to the patient, the cooperation of all members of the health care team is imperative. The nurse who works closely with patients may be aware of areas in which patient teaching is weak or lacking. Suggestions by staff nurses often lead to improvements in every area of nursing, including that of patient teaching.

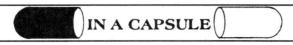 IN A CAPSULE

General purposes of patient teaching include promotion of health, adherence to prescribed regimen, maintenance of independence, provision of basic information, and increased ability to cope with altered lifestyle. Nurses can stress promotion of health to hospitalized patients by teaching measures to prevent recurrence of the current condition and by emphasizing general hygiene.

Patient education is only one means of approaching the complex problem of adherence to prescribed regimen. A greater degree of independence can be attained when the patient accepts any physical limitations and learns to effectively use any special equipment needed. Factual information is one of the first considerations in planning most patient education. The nurse must allow ample time for the patient to practice neces-

sary skills before discharge. Helping the patient to learn to cope with a decreased level of functioning and/or altered life-style may be one of the most difficult patient teaching tasks for the nurse to accomplish.

The nurse is legally responsible for patient education, but all health professionals share this obligation. The nurse is in a key position to promote patient education programs. Collaboration of personnel from various departments in the agency is necessary to establish an effective patient education program. A patient education program cannot function effectively without the cooperation of physicians. The nurse can be instrumental in building a good relationship. Interdisciplinary involvement in the planning and implementation of patient education programs results in maximum benefits for the patient.

DO YOU REMEMBER

- the general purposes of patient education?
- how the nurse can stress health promotion?
- ways in which the nurse can help the patient maintain independence?
- some general areas of basic facts to be included in patient teaching?
- who is legally responsible for patient education?
- why it is essential to have the cooperation of the physician in patient education?

CAN YOU DESCRIBE

- factors that increase patient adherence to the prescribed regimen?
- points of importance in teaching needed skills?
- how the nurse can help the patient to learn to cope with a decreased level of functioning and/or an altered life-style?
- practices that tend to produce a congenial atmosphere in planning a patient education program?
- some approaches the nurse can use to secure greater cooperation of the physician in patient teaching?
- the value of interdisciplinary involvement in patient education?

ACTION, PLEASE

1. Patient adherence to prescribed regimen.

Work in small groups.

You are a part of the nursing team on a medical unit caring for diabetic patients. The head nurse has scheduled a patient care conference. The patient concerned is Carol Lenden, a 19-year-old woman who was diagnosed as diabetic 2 years previously. She was married at age 15 and has one child. Her husband is a truck driver and often out of town for a week at a time. This is the third time this year that Carol has been admitted to the emergency room in diabetic coma. Each time her husband has been out of town.

The purpose of this conference is to determine the reason for Carol's nonadherence to the prescribed diabetic regimen. Role play to attempt to find an answer to the problem. One student can play the part of Carol, one student Carol's husband, and the remainder of students the nurses on the unit.

a. The nursing team meets to try to determine the general approach to use before Carol and her husband join the nurses. Some questions that the nurses might have are: (Add other questions)

Is Carol taking her insulin and adhering to the prescribed diet?
Do you think Carol is trying to get attention from her husband?
Does he oversee Carol's regimen when he is home?

_____

_____

b. Below are some suggested areas of concern to discuss when Carol and her husband join the group. Add other areas of concern to this list.

Knowledge of diabetes
Insulin administration
    Knowledge
    Administration
Motivation for maintaining health

_____

_____

  c. Discuss possible alternatives in reaching some kind of solution to the problem. Carol and her husband can answer questions in any manner and give whatever information desired. The nursing team should produce several approaches to solving the problem.

_____

_____

2. *What Would You Do?* You are a staff nurse on a medical/surgical unit. A doctor who frequently admits patients to the unit is dubious of any nurse's ability to give patients the health information needed and requires a specific order for all patient teaching. You are aware that many of the doctor's patients have learning needs that are not being met during hospitalization.

More than one of the following options is acceptable. Give your rationale for using or rejecting each option.

  a. Give the patient the needed information without asking the doctor's permission.

_____

_____

  b. Report to the doctor any information requested by the patient and ask for suggestions in presenting it.

_____

_____

  c. Prepare an individualized patient teaching plan and present it to the doctor for approval.

_____

_____

  d. Tell the doctor that patient teaching is included in your job description and that you must do it.

_____

_____

What is the next step in providing adequate teaching for this doctor's patients?

_____

_____

_____

7

Special Considerations in Teaching Patients

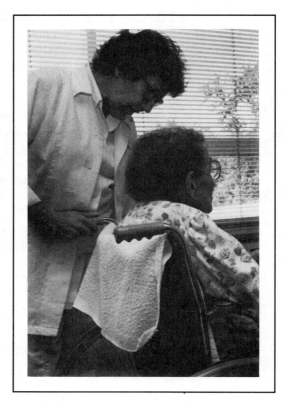

OBJECTIVES

Upon completion of this chapter, the student will be able to:

- state advantages and limitations of informal teaching.
- note the effective use of contract teaching.
- discuss advantages, disadvantages, and special planning for group teaching.
- discuss the necessity of prioritizing learning needs.
- note the impact of a positive approach and patient involvement in teaching.
- compare adaptations of teaching principles and methods in relation to the preschooler, the school-age child, and the adolescent.
- state several general characteristics of adult learners.

The true teacher imparts knowledge at every opportunity.
Anonymous

- discuss differences in approaches to teaching young adults and middle adults.
- describe physiological changes in the elderly that have an impact on learning.
- explain special considerations in teaching the elderly patient.
- list several suggestions for saving time in teaching patients effectively.

GLOSSARY OF TERMS*

Contract teaching   Teaching approach in which both patient and nurse accept responsibilities by signing a contract with goals for each.

Media-based instruction   Presentation of teaching material through the use of audiovisual equipment such as videotapes and computers.

*Definitions applicable to content.

The same teaching/learning principles apply in patient teaching as in any educational situation. There are, however, additional factors that must be considered in teaching patients. The nurse/patient relationship is different from the usual teacher/student contact because the nurse strives to meet the physiological and psychosocial as well as the learning needs of patients. Illness imposes physical limits that are not seen in the usual classroom. The psychosocial factors related to illness often further complicate the teaching process. The wide range of ages of patients requires adaptations in teaching. Each patient is unique and the teaching must be individualized.

GENERAL APPROACHES TO PATIENT TEACHING

The following are not considered teaching strategies but are general methods of approach used by the nurse in patient teaching. Various strategies can be used whether the teaching is formal or informal, individual or group.

Formal/Informal Teaching

When nurses hear the term "patient teaching", the picture of a formal session may come to mind. This chapter is primarily concerned with formal teaching, but a large percentage of patient teaching is informal. There is no detailed assessment process or written plan for informal teaching, but it is an important part of patient teaching. The nurse perceives a learning need and fulfills the need at the time it becomes apparent.

Many nurses do not realize the amount of teaching they do each week. Any time a nurse explains a procedure or tells a patient why a certain medication was ordered, this is informal teaching. Often when a formal teaching plan is ready to be presented, it is found that most of the material has been covered informally. This reduces the time required to implement the formal plan, because a reference to the information already covered is all that is necessary.

Another way nurses teach informally is by role modeling. How can nurses teach good hygienic practices if they ignore these practices? The nurse can teach medical asepsis by using meticulous handwashing practices with casual reference to the reasons during the procedure. Other practices can be a matter of informal conversation during routine hygienic care such as emphasizing the importance of oral hygiene while assisting with morning care.

Nurses should be aware of opportunities for informal teaching but should not repeat information the patient already knows. For example, when assisting a patient in deep breathing and coughing, the nurse should ask if the patient understands the reasons for the procedure before giving an explanation. If the patient is aware of the facts, this is an opportunity for positive reinforcement. The nurse can praise the knowledge and give recognition for previous learning.

Any informal teaching should be documented the same as formal teaching. If there is a need for further teaching on the topic, this should be noted on the chart. Details of documentation will be discussed later.

Contract Teaching

This is sometimes considered a teaching strategy, but it is more of a general approach since various teaching methods may be used. Contract teaching deals with acceptance of responsibilities by both patient and nurse for the teaching/learning process. The learning contract is a tool that formalizes the agreement of the participants to fulfill their responsibilities. It can provide motivation, a means of communication, and standards for evaluation.

Contracting may be threatening to some patients. They may see it as a legal document if the term "contract" is used. Since it requires decision making on the part of the patient, a person lacking in self-confidence might want to avoid this approach. It may seem to be time-consuming on the part of the nurse, but it can save time if the patient will accept the responsibility for learning. It is a certain way to involve the learner in the process and a good way to encourage adherence.

Contract teaching promotes affective learning in that attitudes are changed more readily if the learner views the process as personal accomplishment. For example, if the contract specifies that Mrs. Norris will plan a low-cholesterol diet for a week, the opportunity to include low-cholesterol foods that she likes will give her a sense of satisfaction. Realizing that she can plan the diet and still have food that she enjoys tends to increase acceptance of and adherence to the prescribed regimen.

Contracting is not applicable in all situations. It is not readily adaptable for patients who are hospitalized for short periods. Persons with chronic problems and those who are already motivated to adopt new health habits benefit more from this approach than other patients. A reward at the end of the contract period will make meeting the goal more attractive.

Health care agencies often have their own forms for teaching contracts, but it is no problem to develop one for the individual patient. Sometimes contracts are devised to go with specific standardized teaching plans. These, just as the plans, must be individualized to be effective. Figure 7.1 is a sample of items that might be incorporated into the teaching/learning contract.

Teaching contracts can be written in any manner. Their greatest strength is providing something in writing for patients to see exactly what is expected of them and what they can expect from the nurse. Not all nurses are comfortable with contract teaching and not all patients are willing to cooperate, but it is an approach worth trying.

Teaching/Learning Contract

Learning Need: *Knowledge deficit: Insulin injections*	
Goal: *Prepare and give to self insulin injections*	
Short-Term Goals	Date Completed
Nurse Will: *Demonstrate injection procedure* *Provide equipment for practice* *Spend 10 minutes twice daily supervising practice*	9/2 9/2, 9/4, 9/5 9/2–9/6
Patient Will: *Practice injection procedure 15 minutes four times daily* *Successfully self-inject insulin*	9/2–9/6 9/7
Patient Bonus: *Book of choice from patient education library* If Completed By: *September 10*	
Signatures Patient *Melissa Barnes* Nurse *Charlotte Henry, RN*	Date *Sept 2*

Figure 7.1 Teaching/learning contract

Group Teaching

With the workload of the average nurse, time is too often a factor in the amount of patient teaching that can be done in any given week. Group teaching, which does have some advantages, is one answer to the time factor. Each group session will require more time than an individual session but much less time than multiple one-on-one sessions. All patients scheduled to be in the group must be carefully assessed to determine if they are ready for group teaching. They must have resolved any psychological problems regarding the condition to be able to benefit from a group session.

Group sessions have an advantage in that the patient sees other people who have the same problems. The interchange can be beneficial. Patients who have dealt with the condition for a longer period of time are able to share some solutions to problems and methods of coping that they have worked out over a period of time. The nurse also can gain insights from things that are shared. Sharing feelings in a group can help meet psychological needs of the members.

Group size is a major factor in the effectiveness of group teaching. The group cannot be too large, or some individuals will not actively participate. Small groups of not more than seven are often considered ideal. It can be very effective to have the group plan the goals and activities together in the initial session. The instructor may prefer to have a plan with specific objectives to share with the group at the first meeting. Regardless, there should be a written plan for all to follow. The plan can be expanded or reduced according to the needs of the members. Scheduling can be a problem, since the best time for each member must be considered.

Planning the environment will have an impact on the success of the program. A well-lighted, well-ventilated room that is private and quiet is essential. A table that all participants can be seated around or chairs arranged in a circle allow each member to see the others and feel more like they are part of a "family". Serving coffee, tea, or cold drinks often makes the participants more relaxed. Taking time for the members to get acquainted can establish a general atmosphere for compatibility and sharing of concerns.

The nurse who is instructing the group should play the role of a resource person to as great an extent as possible. This encourages more participation by the members. However, this is not always possible since some topics must have a basic core of information included. Evaluation is more difficult in a group situation. The group situation may be somewhat of a screening process to determine which patients need additional individualized time.

Establishing Priorities

Constraints of Time

Time seems to be a factor in most teaching situations. A common complaint of many classroom instructors is that more time is needed to adequately cover the material. Nurses have this same concern regarding patient teaching. Lack of time is not so much because of duties of the nurse that preclude teaching but the fact that length of hospitalization has shortened dramatically. Many patients are acutely ill during most of their hospital stay and are discharged as soon as they are physiologically stable. There may be little notice regarding the time of discharge. This does not leave adequate time for even initial teaching. Patients may be overwhelmed at the time of discharge with so many instructions that there is no way they can understand all of them.

Reinforcement is essential if teaching is to be effective. Since time is such a crucial factor, the necessity for prioritizing learning needs is emphasized. There must be time available for the patient to practice skills, review factual information, and clarify all concepts. With chronic illnesses, teaching must take place over a period of time. It is started in the hospital setting. However, patients often leave before there is sufficient time for practice. Patients with chronic illnesses must have some kind of follow-up. The hospital nurse can use telephone or written communication to alert outside health personnel to learning needs of the patient as well as teaching that has been initiated.

Prioritizing Needs

When it is known that the patient will be hospitalized for only a short time, planning must be started on admission and learning needs established with the admission interview. This is the time that priorities for teaching should be set. The following information must be determined: Which learning needs are essential for functioning immediately after discharge? Which items can be most effectively taught at a later date? Who or what agency should be alerted at time of discharge to follow up on a teaching program? How should reinforcement be planned for the immediate learning needs? Which areas of knowledge deficit do not relate to the current condition?

Each of these questions must be answered on an individual basis. For example, a patient is admitted with a compound fracture of the right leg. From all appearances, hygienic measures are ignored at home. The nursing history reveals that the patient's diet consists primarily of meat and potatoes with a bit of dessert on the side. The patient's teeth would profit from a trip to a dental hygienist, or even regular brushings. This patient probably will be in the hospital for only a short time. How should patient teaching be prioritized?

Obviously, the first thing that must be considered is care of the injured leg. This teaching must be started immediately and reinforced at every opportunity. Diet or oral hygiene may be the next priority. Nutritional information could be communicated when serving meal trays, with a follow-up at the next meal to determine if the patient retained facts previously presented. Oral hygiene as well as general hygienic measures could be stressed during morning care. Time would be the determining factor in what could be taught. Care of the injured limb is necessary. Teaching in the other areas would be beneficial to the patient.

Other Factors to Consider in Patient Teaching

Positive Approach

Taking a positive approach in patient teaching can lead to more effective results. Assuming that the patient will be a successful learner and that the nurse will be a successful teacher contributes to better results. Attitudes can make or break the outcome of any teaching effort. A person who feels unable to learn probably will not learn. The same is true of the ability to teach. A confident attitude usually leads to desired results.

Joint Endeavor

Patient teaching must be a joint endeavor to be most effective. The nurse should involve the patient in all aspects—assessing the need, establishing the goal, planning the learning activities, and evaluating the outcome. The skillful communicator can enable the patient to arrive at the goal previously identified by the nurse. Often the patient will be the one most able to evaluate how well a concept is understood, a regimen is accepted, or a skill is mastered. But the patient cannot do all of the planning. The nurse must know what the eventual outcome must be and plan accordingly.

ADAPTING TEACHING TO DEVELOPMENTAL LEVEL

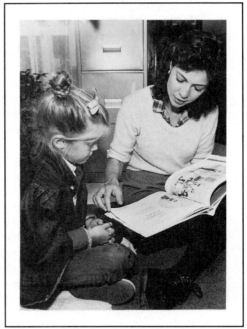

Principles of teaching and learning are considered universally applicable, but special adaptations must be made according to the developmental level of the learner. It is obvious that the same teaching plan could not be used for both a school-age child and an adult. Following are teaching suggestions for various age groups.

Preschoolers

Parent Involvement

The parent is the best person to teach the infant or toddler. The child is accustomed to the tone of voice and directions of the parents. The child as well as the parents are geared to the schedule of routines that are followed at home. Any new routines should be added to those already established with as little change as possible to lessen the trauma to both child and parent. Children benefit from teaching at an early age. For the child 2 to 5 years of age, parents are the primary target of patient teaching. However, children will be more cooperative while hospitalized and after returning home if the teaching is on their level and addressed to them with the parents listening in.

General Approaches in Teaching

Preschoolers are very egocentric. The world revolves around them, and all events are related to them. They like to ask questions, but the nurse must be very careful in giving explanations. Questions should be answered directly and in language preschoolers can understand. Any machines or equipment should be carefully explained. The nurse should let the child try the equipment if possible. Since preschoolers are an energetic and restless group, any teaching sessions should be kept short, 10 to 15 minutes maximum.

Honesty in communication with any age group is important but especially with children in this age group. If the child is told that a procedure will not hurt, only to find out that it does, the credibility of the nurse will be destroyed. The child has some knowledge of anatomy. Any further explanations regarding procedures to be done should be done simply with the use of models and correct anatomical names used for body parts. The child needs to know the reason for the hospitalization and to be reassured that it is not because of misbehavior.

Anticipated surgery needs careful explanations with simple descriptions of what bandages to expect, how much the surgery will hurt, and how it will help the child to feel better after recuperation. The child should be encouraged to tell what has been learned at frequent intervals to ensure that the information is understood. Most preschoolers enjoy displaying their knowledge to family, visitors, and nurses. This provides an opportunity to praise their efforts.

The use of play is one of the most effective adjuncts to teaching that can be used with preschoolers. Toys and dolls can be used with the child playing the part of the doctor or nurse. The nurse can help the child pretend to carry out procedures that the health care team performs while the child is hospitalized. Parents can continue this after discharge.

School-Age Children

Play and Games

School-age children are usually a delight to teach. They are eager to learn and beginning to see relationships between cause and effect. Play is useful during the early school years but is at a more sophisticated level than with the younger child. Coloring books related to anatomy can be fun and are good instructional tools. These years are competitive ones. The child wants to win every game. Creative teaching plans can be constructed in which the child must learn some specific information in order to win. Teaching sessions can be planned to have the child compete against self in ability or time required to perform a procedure. Charts to show progress or stickers to put on a calendar can be an incentive for the child to work hard at mastery.

Teaching Sessions

Teaching materials that are written at a basic level are excellent to use with children in this age group. The material should be left with the child to read and try to comprehend, since this is the approach used at school. The child will usually willingly cooperate. The nurse should check later to ensure that the concepts gained from the reading are correct. Any procedures should be explained directly. The child will usually appreciate a more adult approach. Correct anatomical terms should be used with careful explanations of equipment and procedures. Anatomical models are effective aids.

The child should be included from the beginning in planning teaching. The nurse should explain the general content to be included. The child should be allowed to decide the times to work and set the goals as long as they are acceptable. Since school-age children are accustomed to being in a classroom situation, teaching sessions can be longer than with preschoolers. However, they should not last more than 30 minutes. Parents should be included in any teaching sessions but in a background role. The child should be encouraged to express any fears or concerns regarding the hospital, the health care personnel, or the illness.

Adolescents

There are times when parents feel that adolescents are indeed the most difficult age group with which to deal. These are tumultuous years in which there is a struggle for identity and a battle between independence and the need for support. The peer group is more important than parents or teachers. It is next to impossible to consider all wants and needs of adolescents when planning teaching. A caring attitude is essential, as well as a genuine attempt to understand adolescents' emotional reactions to physical disorders.

Effective Approaches

Since adolescents are struggling toward independence, they should be included in all of the planning. Their opinion should be sought in all aspects of the teaching sessions. Since adolescents are accustomed to 45- to 50-minute classes, teaching sessions can be longer. The nurse and the adolescent should work together in setting realistic goals. Flexibility should be exercised in scheduling and presentations. Contract teaching can be very effective with this age group.

While the parents should be included in any teaching with younger age groups, this may not be advantageous with adolescents. Parents need to be informed of the physical condition of the teenager and specifics of the treatment regimen, but this can be accomplished in separate sessions with them. There are instances when some confidences must be kept in order to maintain the teenager's trust. If the information given in confidence must be divulged for the safety of the patient, the nurse should tell the patient and give specifics as to why it must be told and with whom it will be shared.

The adolescent is ready and able to assimilate a great deal of information. Scientific terms can and should be used but not without explaining each term. Adolescents even more than school-age children will profit from literature to review between teaching sessions. The nurse should be available to answer any questions they might have and should answer these questions as openly and honestly as possible. If the nurse cannot give an adequate answer, another member of the health care team should be found to answer the question. Adolescents appreciate full explanations and are more likely to adhere to regimens when the alternatives and consequences are explained. They are oriented to the present, and immediate advantages are more meaningful than long-term results.

Body Image

Adolescents are very aware of body image. Any condition that will have an effect on their physical appearance requires sensitivity. For example, if the loss of hair following chemotherapy will be a problem, they should be taught about the use of wigs and hats. Different applications of makeup that will hide facial scars can be explored. They should be taught about the healing process of any incision and the length of time the scar may remain visible. Role identity is somewhat related to body image. Any diagnosis that has a possibility of altering identity, such as an orthopedic injury of an athlete, must be treated with the same caring attitude and understanding as a change of body image.

Since peers are the strongest influence on adolescents, they should be allowed to invite some of their peers to teaching sessions if desired. These sessions could include some information about general health maintenance so that the teaching will benefit the patient and friends in their daily lives.

CHECK IT OUT

Think back to your adolescent years and try to answer the following questions.

What was your attitude toward adults in general and teachers in particular?

What were some of your favorite classes in school? Was this related more to the subject material or to the teacher?

What classroom approaches provided the strongest stimulus for your best efforts?

What behaviors of the teachers did you find most distasteful?

From your responses to these questions, add to the preceding discussion about adolescent learners and indicate areas with which you agree or disagree.

Adult Learners

Many nurses deal primarily with adult patients, which cover a span from 20 years of age on. Adulthood may be divided into three phases: the young adult, from 20 to 40 years of age; middle adulthood, from 40 to 60 years of age; and the elderly years, starting at age 60. The elderly group is sometimes subdivided, since there is quite a difference between the average 60- and 90-year old person. To a young person, 40 years of age is often considered the peak and the rest of life a downward slide. However, many people over age 40 will disagree. Age tends to be relative. All statements made are generalizations that cannot be applied to every person in a specific age bracket. They are guidelines only. Teaching adult patients in a manner that will enable them to retain and apply the information is often a challenge.

General Characteristics of Adult Learners

The following are general premises that are typical of many but not all adult learners. There is a blurring of abilities and responses in chronological age groups. Patients must be assessed individually. For example, some 70-year-old persons are as capable as others in their fifties.

1. Activities that maintain or increase self-esteem tend to act as secondary motivators. Adults are accustomed to making decisions and view self-direction in learning situations as a boost to self-esteem.

2. Adults tend to take errors personally. They believe that having to be corrected or being unable to grasp a concept immediately is a reflection on their ability, which acts to lower their self-esteem.

3. Adults need to be able to integrate new ideas into their current knowledge. They have a stockpile of life experiences, which serves as a learning resource.

4. Any new information that conflicts with previous knowledge forces a reevaluation of prior learning. This impedes the learning process in that assimilation of the new material is slowed.

5. Unusual learning tasks may cause anxiety, which acts as a barrier to learning.

6. Adults, especially the older group, may be slower in learning psychomotor skills but may compensate by attempting to be extremely accurate in any procedure.

7. Adult learners tend to prefer a straightforward how-to approach. They are more attuned to the immediate application of knowledge.

8. A comfortable learning environment is essential for adult learners. Adults learn most readily in a psychological environment that is informal and friendly, one in which they feel valued as individuals. A comfortable physical environment is a must for learning to take place.

9. Items highest on adults' list of irritations in the teaching/learning situation are long sessions and absent or insufficient practice or learning time.

Young Adults

The early adult years, from age 20 to 40 years, are viewed by most persons as a time when there is plenty of energy for tasks to be accomplished. These are the childbearing years and are considered to be fruitful in many other aspects. Except for the early twenties, when many young adults are in college, this is not generally considered a learning period. Teaching adults, especially 30- to 40-year-old adults, is approached in a different manner than teenagers or college students.

The young adult learner needs a practical reason for learning. With all of the other activities going on in the lives of people in this age group, there must be a good reason for spending time and energy in learning something new. Young adults too often take good health for granted. The formulation of mutually acceptable goals may be one of the most important aspects in teaching this age group. They must see a need for the new information or skills. If need is established, people in this age group present no problems in the teaching/learning process. They often have young children, and parents will do anything that enables them to maintain a level of functioning that allows for care of the children.

Middle Adults

The period from 40 to 60 years of age differs from earlier adulthood. These individuals are more aware of possible health problems than young adults. This is often seen as a period when productivity has come to an end, the mind is less fruitful, and new tasks cannot be learned. This could not be further from the truth. Many adults in this age group are more active and capable of learning than previously, when as parents they were preoccupied with child rearing. Others, however, may lack self-confidence, which can cause avoidance of the risk of failure in learning anything new. Rather than take this risk, learning activities are avoided for one reason or another. The nurse must approach patient teaching with individuals who lack self-confidence at a simple level and praise each small victory.

Preferred Approaches. Middle adults have a broad base of knowledge, so new information needs to be presented in such a manner that it can be easily integrated with known facts. Any information that conflicts with concepts they consider a truth must be reevaluated. Thus it is integrated more slowly with the held beliefs.

With this age group, individuals tend to view errors as a direct affront to their self-esteem. Since self-esteem is a strong secondary motivator for adult learners, this is a point that needs particular caution in teaching. Any misconceptions should be gently corrected. It should be pointed out that other people have the same difficulties.

Some adults may be a bit slower in mastering new skills, but they are quite capable of learning complex procedures. Individuals who have worked with their hands throughout their lifetime may be able to master, for example, giving injections better than the average younger person. Some patients in this age group may welcome a media-based approach to instruction. However, many will be cautious regarding this unfamiliar approach.

People in this age group like a direct approach to learning. It is true that they need the rationale for doing things in a particular way, but a straightforward method can be very effective. They must be a part of planning sessions and goal setting. Most middle adults have set goals for themselves through the years and have met the majority of them. If the teaching goals are accepted by the patient, the chances for meeting them are greater.

Irritations. There are some things that middle adults find especially irritating. Long sessions tend to become exasperating for them. They require sufficient practice time for mastery of skills or assimilation of information. They also want private practice periods, but the nurse should not allow extensive practice without some observation since mistakes practiced too long are very difficult to correct.

A comfortable learning environment is a must. This includes psychological as well as physical comfort. A physically comfortable environment is easily arranged. The nurse can create a comfortable psychological environment, but this must be started well in advance of the actual teaching session. Early establishment of rapport is the first step. A calm attitude that expresses caring sets the stage for effective teaching. A thorough educational assessment with identification of specific learning needs reduces teaching time. Middle adults resent the repetition of information well known to them.

Elderly Learners

As the percentage of the population over 65 years of age increases, nurses will be caring for more patients in this age group. Most of the items noted for the adult learner are applicable to the elderly, but there are some additional considerations. The nurse must be aware of the person's past experiences in order to relate them to current problems and goals. It is important that the patient have input into the teach-

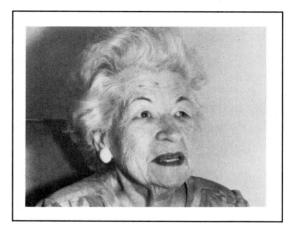

ing process. It may be very difficult to motivate the elderly. Some may feel that it is hardly worth the effort to learn new information and skills since they think their life is nearing the end. The nurse can help motivate the patient to learn by showing how the acquisition of new skills will increase the quality of life, even though the quantity may be limited.

Effect of Physiological Changes

There are a number of physiological changes that accompany aging. Three of these that are most likely to have an impact on learning are vision, hearing, and reaction time. As the eyes age, there is a loss of elasticity, pupils become smaller and react more slowly, the incidence of cataracts increases, and color perception becomes less acute.

Physiological changes result in a gradual decline in hearing in most individuals, creating problems with pitch, volume, and rate of speech. Acuity is lost for the higher pitch, with lower tones being more readily heard. Rapid speech can become unintelligible since the elderly person tends to require more time to perceive the stimulus, to translate the meaning, and to act on it. Hearing loss tends to cause more withdrawal and sense of isolation than other physiological changes.

Neural transmission slows and reaction time increases in the elderly. This varies in individuals and sometimes seems to be related to habit. A manner of reacting slowly can become a general personality characteristic even before a person reaches these years. There is no doubt that there is a slowing of reaction time with aging. This has many implications for patient teaching, especially regarding methods of presenting materials. It also increases the amount of safety measures that should be included in patient teaching.

Environmental Arrangements

Providing an environment conducive to learning requires special attention. Some of the physiological changes noted may be seen at an earlier age, but most will be present to some degree in nearly every individual past 70 years of age. To compensate for visual changes, rooms should be brightly lighted with no glare. Any visual aids must have large, well-spaced letters with primary colors, which are more readily distinguished. If teaching a group, seats must be arranged so that all participants are reasonably close to any visual materials. The nurse must make sure that any patients who wear glasses have these available and that the lenses are clean.

To compensate for hearing deficiencies that often accompany aging, elimination of extraneous noises is most beneficial. The nurse should face the learner and avoid covering the mouth for any reason. The rate of speech should be slower, and lower voice tones should be used in all teaching. The female nurse might use a bright red lipstick to facilitate speechreading. When speaking to a group of patients, a microphone can be helpful but should be properly adjusted to eliminate any static. The audience should always be asked how well they can hear. The nurse should be aware of nonverbal indicators that words are not clearly heard or understood, such as learning forward, cupping hands to ears, frowning while attempting to hear, or starting separate conversations. If any patients have hearing aids, batteries may need to be checked.

Elderly persons need more frequent breaks than younger persons. They should not be expected to remain seated for more than 20 or 30 minutes without a break. Remember that one of the physiological changes accompanying age is reduced kidney function. This, with the frequent use of diuretics, decreases the length of time between trips to the bathroom. These breaks also give the individuals an opportunity to exercise stiff joints, thus stimulating circulation.

Some elderly persons tend to prefer solitary learning, but this is not true of all. The desire to learn can be stimulated by the presence of others. A small group can dispel some of the loneliness, and a feeling of camaraderie is often established within the group. Many elderly persons readily form new bonds with others for the companionship afforded.

Memory

A problem often noted in cognitive functioning in the elderly is memory, especially short-term memory. It is too often assumed that older people cannot remember facts. There is some deterioration in memory with age, but the loss is considered minor until 85 years and older. Problems seem to be primarily with meaningless learning, complex learning, and new information that requires reassessment of old learning. Meaningless material is poorly retained, since there is no reason or motivation to learn it. Complex material plus any distractions during learning make the process difficult. Elderly persons have accumulated large stores of information, and scanning for recall takes longer.

Suggestions to improve short-term memory for the elderly, which may be applicable to younger groups, include the following.

1. New information should be meaningful, be related to past knowledge, and be accompanied by aids to organize the material.
2. Information should be presented at a rate that allows ample time for mastery.
3. Only one idea should be presented at a time.
4. All material should be summarized frequently.
5. Feedback should be used frequently to validate understanding.

The elderly are quite capable of learning, even though the rate is slowed, especially in the 80- and 90-year-old group. They can learn new techniques and will be motivated to do so if it is a factor in maintaining independence. A summary of points covered at the end of each session with a written account or a tape for the visually impaired to review before the next session can be very helpful.

The use of terminology familiar to the elderly patient is critical. The nurse should become acquainted with the colloquialisms they have used since youth and describe functions with the use of these whenever possible. Written handouts with clear pictures and simple words can be beneficial. All teaching sessions with the elderly must be well organized, be slow paced, and progress from simple to complex. Any new material must be tied to old concepts to be meaningful to the elderly. If new information can be interrelated with the old, these people have little trouble assimilating it.

Information about medications is essential in teaching the elderly. They need to know what each tablet or liquid is for, when it should be taken, and any side effects. An item often overlooked is instructions regarding what to do if a dosage is missed. Some may think that doubling up for several days missed will prevent any problems. This misconception must be corrected. A problem may be in forgetting when medications were taken. There are many commercial containers available for organizing a week's supply of medications with each tablet or tablets in a special time slot for each day of the week. The elderly may need a guide to help in placing each week's supply in the proper slots. A diagram can be made showing the colors and shapes of each tablet, along with the name of the medication that appears on the bottle. The elderly patient needs written instructions regarding the medications. These need to be in large print with a picture of the tablet and very specific directions.

TIMELY TEACHING TIPS

Stretching Teaching Time There is little anyone can do about time, but time can be used wisely to accomplish the things that are most important. There are numerous ways in which patient teaching time can be stretched. Standard teaching plans serve as a guideline that can be adapted to the individual patient. Group instruction is another method that can be used in selected situations.

Audiovisual Aids The use of audiovisual aids can be a time saver. It is sometimes said that one picture is worth a thousand words. A diagram to illustrate the teaching content is a good example. The nurse can explain in simple terms the pathophysiology of a hiatal hernia. It can be done in half the time with an illustration. Films can show techniques of simple procedures or more complicated ones such as colostomy care.

Caution in the use of audiovisual aids has been noted. They should not be relied on as the only means of giving information to the patient. All adjuncts must be carefully screened. Written material must be at the proper level. All audiovisual materials must be accurate and must contain the facts the nurse wants to present. Audiovisual aids make excellent springboards for discussion but should not be used without a short preparatory session with the patient and followed up by discussion and further teaching.

Time Saving Documentation Although it is more often considered time-consuming, documentation can actually save nurses time. It can be used to promote team effort in patient teaching. The notation of what has been covered eliminates repetition of the same material. Checklists are an excellent method of keeping up with teaching progress. A simple list of areas to be covered in patient teaching can be prepared with each member of the health care team checking items that have been presented to the patient.

Take Advantage of Each Opportunity Teaching should start when the patient is admitted. This allows maximum time for patient teaching and identifies learning needs from the first day of admission. To provide the patient with adequate information and skills to adequately care for self following discharge, it is necessary to teach at every opportunity, as mentioned in the section on informal teaching. Mealtime lends itself to dietary teaching, whether regarding a special diet or normal balanced nutrition. Bath time is an excellent time not only for assessment but also for emphasizing general hygienic measures, oral hygiene, skin care, and any pertinent points regarding foot care. Administering medications presents a good opportunity to give and to reinforce information about medications the patient is taking. These are only a few instances during routine care when the nurse can teach the patient.

Time Saving Language Another factor that will actually save time is to speak the patient's language and be specific in all instructions. This may seem strange to note as a time saver, but explanations that are understandable only have to be given once. There will be fewer questions when the patient understands what has been explained.

Key Points First An additional approach to increase understanding is to place the key points in the first part of any presentation. Listeners tend to remember to a greater degree information that is included in the first part of any communication. Verbal headings can be placed in the material. What is about to follow can be stated, such as, "Let's talk about the type of exercise you will need to do." As with all areas of nursing, students develop an approach of their own. Some of these suggestions may be helpful, while others may not seem natural. Students may develop approaches that are superior to those presented and may wish to share their ideas with others.

IN A CAPSULE

Teaching plans represent a *formal* approach, but *informal teaching* is equally important. A *teaching/learning contract* specifies responsibilities of both participants. *Group teaching* can be effective with careful assessment and selection of participants and definitive planning.

The nurse must *establish priorities* if time is a crucial factor in patient teaching. Teaching is best approached in a *positive* manner as a *joint endeavor.* Teaching must be *adapted to the developmental level* of the learner.

The *preschooler* must be answered honestly, but the parents are the primary learners. The use of play is one of the most effective methods of teaching this age group. Materials written at a basic level and competitive approaches appeal to the *school-age child.* The child should be the central figure in all teaching activities with parents assuming a background role. *Adolescents* should be included in the planning and allowed flexibility in scheduling with the teaching oriented to the present. Parents are not always included in the teaching. Conditions affecting body image must be approached with sensitivity.

Some of the *general characteris-*

tics of the adult learner are related to self-esteem. Information coherent with previous knowledge is most readily assimilated. Adults prefer a straightforward approach in a comfortable environment. *Young adults*, from 20 to 40 years of age, tend to take good health for granted but are enthusiastic learners when a need is perceived. *Middle adults*, from 40 to 60 years of age, are more aware of potential health problems and are receptive to learning. They tend to be averse to long sessions and insufficient practice time. They prefer to be a part of the planning.

There are additional considerations in teaching the *elderly learner.* Physiological changes require adaptations for visual and hearing deficiencies. Elderly patients are capable of learning, but the rate is often slowed.

Time savers in teaching include the appropriate use of audiovisual material and group teaching with patient teaching begun on admission and continued at every opportunity.

DO YOU REMEMBER

- the role of informal teaching?
- the importance of establishing teaching priorities?
- general characteristics of the adult learner?
- factors that enhance or decrease learning in young and middle adults?
- physiological changes accompanying aging that have an impact on learning?

CAN YOU DESCRIBE

- what is meant by contract teaching?
- advantages and limitations of group teaching?
- variations in approaches when teaching preschoolers, school-age children, and adolescents?
- adaptations that provide an environment conducive to learning for the elderly?
- tips that save time in teaching?

ACTION, PLEASE

1. Talk with an elderly person, preferable over 80 years of age, with whom you are well acquainted. Determine the amount of visual and auditory deficiencies. Explain to the person that you are trying an experiment.

    a. If there is an auditory deficit:

        Talk in high tones, then low tones.

        Talk rapidly, then slowly.

        Talk facing the person, then with your back turned.

    Under which circumstances could the individual best understand you?

How does this compare with the discussion of the elderly learner?

_____

_____

b. If there is a visual deficit:
   Give the person a short paragraph to read.
      Place the page so that there is a glare on it.
      Stand so that you are blocking the light, then move.
   Make two simple pages with a short-worded message or a simple picture.
      Use red and blue on one page and green and purple on the other.

What response was there to the glare on the page?

_____

_____

What was the reaction to your standing in the light?

_____

_____

Which colors were most readily distinguishable?

_____

_____

How did the reactions compare with the recommendations in the chapter regarding environmental considerations for the elderly?

_____

_____

After trying these approaches, tell your friend the details of your experiment. How will this be applicable to your patient teaching?

_____

_____

2. How Would You Point Out Mistakes to This Patient? Mrs. Fielding is a 50-year-old obese patient who has had gastric stapling to aid in weight reduction. She has been accustomed to eating three large, high-calorie meals a day, but says she never eats between meals. In reinforcing the dietitian's instructions, you have asked the patient to prepare a menu for a week for a balanced diet with six small meals a day. Mrs. Fielding's menu listed three fairly large meals a day with high-calorie snacks between.

More than one response is acceptable. For each option, give the rationale for using or not using it with reference to the application to this age group.

a. "Let's look again at the list the dietitian gave you and see if the calories can be reduced."

_____

_____

b. "These between-meal snacks contain too many calories."

_____

_____

c. "Well, you'll never lose any weight on this diet."

_____

_____

d. "This has some good ideas but may need a few changes."

_____

_____

What would be your response? You may chose one of the above, add to one of them, or use a different approach.

_____

_____

_____

8

The Nurse's Application of the Teaching Process

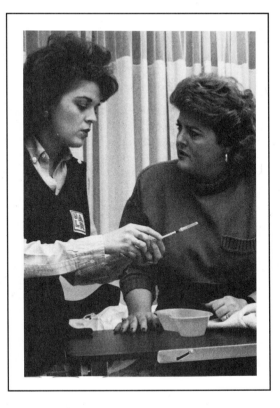

The more you practice what you know, the more you know what to practice. **W. Jenkins**

OBJECTIVES

Upon completion of this chapter, the student will be able to:

- compare the steps in the nursing process and the teaching process.
- identify factors that should be included in an educationally focused patient assessment.
- select applicable nursing diagnoses.
- indicate the importance of well-written goals in patient teaching.
- discuss resources and support systems to be considered in planning patient teaching.
- note factors affecting the selection of content, teaching strategies, and adjuncts.
- describe methods, timing, and manner of evaluating learning.
- document a patient teaching session

to include all essential information.
- give advantages and cautions in the use of standard teaching plans.
- implement an individualized plan for patient teaching in the clinical situation.

*Definitions applicable to content.

Teaching/learning principles have been briefly considered for the purpose of applying them to the process of patient education. The application embodies the steps used in the nursing process. (This can be linked to a learning principle in that the new knowledge is related to past knowledge of the nursing process.) Patient teaching should be an outgrowth of nursing care plans in which learning needs are identified.

THE TEACHING PROCESS

The application readily follows the format of the nursing process. The nursing process points to the individual needs and problems of the patient, and the teaching process emphasizes individualization. Each step in the teaching process from assessment through evaluation with possible revisions will be considered. One further step—documentation of patient teaching—will be included. Aspects of physical care of the patient are documented routinely, but sometimes patient teaching is not as fully documented as it should be. The steps in the teaching process, like those in the nursing process, must all be linked for the teaching process to hold together. If any one step is omitted, the process falls apart.

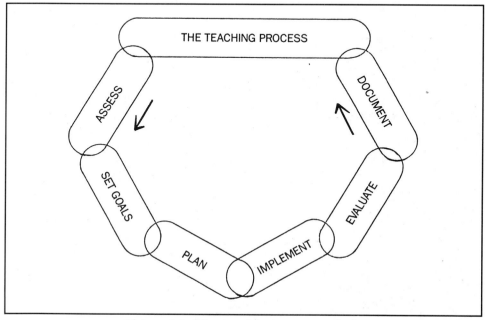

Figure 8.1 The teaching process chain

Patient Assessment

Assessment is the first link of the teaching process chain. It is the systematic collection of data to identify the learning needs of patients as well as any correct or incorrect knowledge. The assessment phase in patient teaching necessarily covers more than the physiological assessment of the patient. It is an educationally focused assessment. In it factors relating to the learning abilities of the patient as well as external factors that have an influence on the teaching/learning process must be considered. It includes the patient's current knowledge and skills as compared with those necessary for independent functioning after discharge.

Factors Affecting the Ability to Communicate

While patient teaching is a form of goal-oriented communication, both participants must communicate for teaching to be effective. The patient's ability to communicate must be assessed in order for the nurse to adequately plan an effective teaching approach. The factors influencing communication discussed in Unit I, Nurse-Patient Communication, are applicable to patient teaching.

The *age and developmental level* of the learner influence the teaching approach, the language usage, and any printed materials used. Because there may be a discrepancy in the chronological and the developmental age, the teaching should be gauged to the developmental age. An adult who is mentally retarded or a child who is a slow learner and reads at a low level will need material that is understandable at the developmental level. On the other hand, some children are able to comprehend material above their chronological age level.

The patient's *social/cultural background* has an impact on language usage and general information included in the teaching. For example, if a patient's religious belief dictates a vegetarian diet, a balanced diet without meat must be formulated. Terminology must be within the framework of the patient's accustomed speech. There may be situations in which the cultural background tends to make a male patient averse to a female teacher or a male patient dislike having a male nurse. The factors must be determined on an individual basis and any adjustments made before any patient teaching is attempted.

The patient's *level of education* has an influence on language usage, but this is not the only determinant. *Language skills* must be assessed. A high school education does not assure language fluency and in some cases does not assure functional literacy. Only by talking with a person can the nurse determine the level of language usage and verbal ability. Many adults are unable to read fluently. Any written material given to these persons for reference will not be of any use. The nurse can surmount this obstacle with a bit of ingenuity and a few simple drawings. It should never be assumed that any patient understands technical terms. When using a medical term, the nurse should ask if it is understood.

Learning Readiness

Individuals can possess the mental capacity, have an advanced education, and appear on the surface to be an ideal learner. However, there may be factors interfering with the learning process that make attempts at teaching futile. Assessing readiness to learn can save time and energy and decrease frustration on the part of both patient and nurse.

The *level of energy* of the patient must be considered. Learning requires an expenditure of energy, as any student will agree. Intense studying can be exhausting. Patients who are very ill, physically weak, or in the early stages of recovering from surgery often do not have enough energy to absorb any new facts. Teaching should not be attempted at this point. After determining that the patient is physically capable, the ability to sit in a chair or walk should be assessed. There are times when teaching should be done with the patient in bed because a walk to another area or sitting in a chair in the room would expend the energy needed for learning.

The *attitude* of patients is an important factor in readiness to learn. This is linked with motivation and mutually acceptable goals, as well as cultural influences. Does the patient accept the need to learn new skills or acquire additional knowledge? Is the nurse viewed as an adequate teacher? The patient may not consider a female nurse to be a capable instructor. A patient may deny the existence of an illness and refuse instruction. The patient may simply resist all efforts directed toward teaching, and the nurse may not be able to determine the cause.

The *anxiety level* of the patient must be assessed. If the health problem is very serious and/or newly diagnosed, the patient's learning capacity will be low. There may be personal problems that are very distracting that block teaching efforts. Assessing the nonverbal communication may give the nurse the key to emotional stresses that can interfere with learning.

The attention span of patients is a factor in any teaching/learning situation. The patient's attention span may always be short, or there may be a particular cause for it at this time. It may be related to anxiety or the current physical *comfort* status. Pain, hunger, and sleepiness will affect the patient's attention span. The patient's status should be determined by direct questions. A teaching session can always be postponed until after lunch, a short nap, or a trip to the restroom. Any time the patient's attention seems to be wandering during a teaching session, it is best to discontinue and go back at a later time. To try to force teaching at this time is a waste of effort for both participants.

Sensory Status

The sensory status of the patient must be assessed before planning teaching approaches. If there are visual deficits, large print and the use of verbal explanations are necessary. Visual components are emphasized when there is a hearing deficit. Motor ability must be taken into account in teaching skills. Injuries or arthritic conditions may restrict full use of hands or extremities. Some special adaptations were discussed in Chapter 7 regarding the elderly patient. These suggestions are applicable to any age patient. It must be remembered that the presence of sensory deficits is not limited to the elderly.

Learning Needs

The assessments in the preceding paragraphs deal with the general status of the patient and related factors to be considered in planning teaching. Assessments to determine the patient's current knowledge must also be carried out.

The nurse must assess the amount of *background knowledge* of the condition that the patient has. It is unnecessary to repeat what the patient already knows. The best way to determine this is by direct questioning. For example, "Tell me what you know about peptic ulcers," would be a start for gaining this information. Any misconceptions could be corrected and any gaps in the knowledge supplied. Further facts about the related anatomy and physiology might help the patient to better understand the dysfunction.

General *health maintenance knowledge* should be considered. Even though it does not seem directly related to the current condition, the nurse should take advantage of any opportunity for stressing maintenance of health and prevention of illness. Every patient can benefit from knowledge of normal nutritional requirements, hygienic practices, and preventive measures. Teaching in these areas is a part of the nurse's responsibilities. Some general health knowledge, such as nutrition, rest, and activity patterns, may be related to the recommended regimen following discharge.

The nurse must assess the specific *skills needed* for care following discharge. These may be simple skills, such as a sitz bath, or skills that require practice by the patient, such as injections, irrigations, or dressings. The nurse should not take the patient's word that a skill has been mastered but should observe the patient carrying out the procedure. The technique may be adequate, or there may be errors that need to be corrected.

If the patient will need follow-up care after discharge in various health agencies, the nurse should assess *the ability to utilize health facilities and services.* Information may be needed on how to make appointments, which facilities are available, and which ones are best for special services. If home care is needed, the patient or family will need to know how to arrange for this. Social workers usually take the responsibility for arranging these services, but the nurse should make certain that someone will be working with the patient after discharge.

A suggested format for the patient assessment portion of a teaching plan is noted in Table 8.1, with a summary of items to be included in each section. Other sections of a teaching plan format will be noted at the end of each discussion section.

Patient Assessment

Factors Affecting Ability to Communicate	Learning Readiness	Sensory Status	Learning Needs
Age/Developmental Level	Energy Level	Visual	Knowledge of Condition
Social/Cultural Background	Anxiety Level	Auditory	General Health Maintenance Knowledge
Level of Education	Comfort	Motor	
Language Skills		Ability	Ability to Use Health Services and Facilities

Table 8.1: Patient assessment.

The patient assessment is fundamental in formulating a teaching plan. The data collected are analyzed to determine the most appropriate approach to teaching. The content to be included is determined by the learning needs assessed. The strategy and language level is colored by the patient's background, level of education, and language skills. The sensory status of the patient has an impact on the strategy and adjuncts used. The learning readiness is of prime importance in setting the time for teaching sessions. Without an adequate patient assessment, it is impossible to individualize patient teaching.

Nursing Diagnosis

Sometimes the nursing diagnosis is separated from the assessment to give it added emphasis. It can be considered a part of assessment, since it is a natural outcome of the assessment. It is the analysis of the facts and briefly describes results of the assessment process. Accepted nursing diagnoses include knowledge deficit, which directly relates to learning, and others such as noncompliance and self-care deficit, which are closely related. Many other nursing diagnosis may be related and become apparent during the course of assessment for patient teaching.

Goal Setting

Goal setting is sometimes included in planning because it shows the direction of the process. Goals and objectives are essentially the same thing. Both indicate a desired end to be reached. Although some prefer terms such as expected outcome or desired outcome, all of the terms indicate the same thing. Goals in the teaching/learning situation should have the same essential components as communication goals. They must be mutually acceptable, be realistic, be measurable, be patient centered, have a time frame, and preferably be written.

(Who) +	Does +	What +	How +	When =	Goal
(Patient)	Recall	Signs/Symptoms Wound Infection	Orally	Tomorrow	
(Patient)	Demonstrate	Dressing Change	Unassisted	By discharge	

Figure 8.2: Components of a goal.

Goal setting serves several related purposes. It is an activity in which both patient and nurse should participate. The discussion and setting of goals can be a factor in helping the patient realize the learning need. After completing the assessment, the nurse should have identified what the patient wants and/or needs to learn. This simplifies mutual acceptance of goals. Goals also act as guides for evaluation at the end of the teaching process.

Mutually Acceptable Goals

Most patients will accept all suggestions, but some may not agree with all of the goals the nurse has presented. For example, the learning need may be related to a weight-reduction diet. The nurse has set a goal for patient adherence to a diet 7 days a week for a weight loss of 2 pounds per week. The patient does not want to stay on the diet 7 days a week. A mutually agreeable goal might involve further reduction of calories 5 days a week with an increase the other 2 days. According to caloric requirements, this should still produce a 2-pound a week loss. This goal could not be evaluated during the average hospital stay but represents a compromise.

Realistic Goals

Goals must specify an outcome that the patient can reasonably be expected to achieve. For a patient who is adapting to a colostomy, a goal stating that the patient will be able to care for self within a week is more than should be expected. Setting several short-term goals will help the patient to realize small successes. The first goal might be to assist the nurse in irrigations, or it could be related to dietary modifications. The goal must be realistic or the patient will not be interested in putting forth any effort toward accomplishment.

Measurable Goals

Setting measurable goals automatically determines a means of evaluation. Goals that deal with the affective domain are difficult to state and to measure. How is acceptance or understanding measured? There must be visible components by which to measure. Acceptance of a colostomy can be measured by the patient's learning efforts in caring for it and any communication regarding future plans.

Many teaching/learning goals are best if broken down into subgoals. A procedure may have several components that can be learned one step at a time. For example, this could be written as follows.

Demonstrate ability to self-inject insulin prior to discharge by completing the following steps.

1. Accurately withdraw specified amounts of solution into insulin syringe.
2. Cleanse area and inject solution into orange or other object.
3. Correctly prepare and self-inject insulin into selected sites three times.

Noting the subgoals tells the patient exactly what is expected and sets the stage for several small successes.

Patient-Centered Goals

Goals in a teaching plan must state what the patient will accomplish. Nursing goals are set, but these are things the nurse wants to accomplish. In contract teaching, for example, there are certain goals for the patient and other goals for the nurse. The goals state the terms of the contract. In all patient teaching, the patient learning goals and the teaching goals of the nurse are closely intertwined.

Time Frame of Goals

The time frame of goals in patient teaching may be changed if progress indicates that the patient will not be able to meet the goal within the time first specified. The primary purpose of a goal is to have something to aim for. The time frame must be a reasonable one, just as the goal must be reasonable.

Written Goals

Teaching/learning goals are best if written. Although informal teaching will not have written goals since it is not planned ahead, the nurse will have a goal in mind.

Formal teaching usually has written goals. These can be given to the patient before the teaching is begun so that both participants know what is expected. Written goals help other health team members determine what teaching is planned. The documentation reveals what has been taught, which promotes team effort in patient teaching.

Nursing Diagnoses	Goals

If more than one nursing diagnosis included in plan, signify with A. or B.	If there are subgoals, list under the primary goal as a. or b.
	Refer goals to a specific nursing diagnosis if more than one: A. _____
	              a.
	              b.
	          B. _____

Table 8.2: Nursing diagnosis and goals.

Planning Considerations

As with the nursing process, planning is the next step in the teaching/learning process. It is an important link in the teaching process chain. Plans must be made to meet the individual patient's learning needs and must stem from the mutually accepted goals. Planning involves a check of the resources available, consideration of the support systems, determination of content, selection of teaching strategy, arrangement of time, and adaptation of all factors to the individual.

Resources

The physical space available must be considered. The teaching may take place in the patient's room. If the patient is in a semiprivate room, it may be advisable to arrange for another space for teaching or select a time when the roommate is out of the room. If more than one patient is to be included or if several family members will be present, arrangements must be made to use a conference room or classroom.

The nurse must assess the teaching adjuncts available, such as any written or audiovisual materials. Health care agencies with strong patient education programs usually have materials written specifically for the lay person on most common diagnoses. These are excellent for most patients but must be previewed by the nurse to determine appropriateness for each particular patient.

Materials written as teaching aids are written primarily for adults and must be adapted for children. The material would also have to be adapted for a patient with a sensory deficit, but the information included serves as an excellent guide. For patients who cannot read, the nurse may need to make simple diagrams to accompany verbal explanations.

The use of audiovisual equipment and any equipment needed to demonstrate procedures must be scheduled and any supplies needed obtained. Supplies are not usually a problem. They are available on the unit, and the cost of many is minimal. If other members of the health team are to be included in the teaching session, arrangements must be made with them.

Support Systems

The nurse must consider the patient's support system, such as family members who are to be included in the teaching sessions. The nurse should assess how much they will participate in care of the patient after discharge. Times must be arranged when the family or friends will be able to attend. Their willingness and ability must also be assessed. Sometimes home care needs to be arranged through an agency if family members are not able or willing to take responsibility for care.

Another support system to consider is that of the nurse. Hospital policies may have an effect on what the nurse is permitted to teach. The nurse may be allowed a certain amount of time for preparation and presentation. The cooperation of personnel from other departments in assisting must be considered. The support of the physician is essential. Legal support is not usually a problem, but the nurse should be careful to fully document teaching, including patient response. As a student nurse, the wisest course of action is to ask the primary nurse or head nurse before beginning any patient teaching, preferably submitting a plan for approval.

Planning Considerations

Resources Needed	Available/ Arrangements	Patient's Support System	Nurse's Support System
Physical space Learning aids needed	Any arrangements Those on hand; need to secure; schedule use; need to be made	Family members who will be involved in care at home. Any necessary scheduling	Institutional policies Physician support Time allowed Primary/head nurse approval
Other health team members	Schedule time		

Table 8.3: Planning considerations.

Plan of Presentation

Selection of Content

The selection of content is highly individualized and based on the assessment. The material will depend in part on the patient's current knowledge. With some patients, little additional information will be needed. Others will need teaching beginning with the basics. The nurse should determine the amount of information the patient has regarding the topic before outlining the content to be included. Establishment of learning needs dictates to an extent the content that will be included in the teaching plan.

For example, an RN is preparing a teaching plan for Mrs. Worth, who is hospitalized with peptic ulcers. In the patient assessment, it is found that her husband had ulcer problems about 5 years ago. Mrs. Worth was included in the patient teaching at that time. Through questioning, it is determined that she is knowledgeable regarding the pathophysiology, predisposing factors, and signs and symptoms of ulcers. Her primary knowledge deficit is related to medications. The selection of content, therefore, would relate more to medications. Notation should be made regarding her knowledge of the condition.

The amount of material presented may be limited by the time available for teaching. Often nurses attempt to overload patients with information. Too many details can confuse the patient and cause a blocking out of the central ideas. Carefully thought out plans with effective visual aids can present a concept at a basic level, where it is easily understood. Outlining the material briefly in a logical sequence makes the session move smoothly and assures that the main points are covered.

Choosing Teaching Strategies and Adjuncts

Various teaching strategies and approaches have been examined. Some techniques and their general application are summarized briefly as follows.

Lecture should be reserved for use with a group.

Discussion is an effective method to impart factual information.

Demonstration is essential in teaching procedures.

Play is very effective with children.

Role play and games are useful tools in special cases but are time-consuming.

Programmed instruction can be utilized only with selected patients.

Instructional aids should be incorporated with all approaches. Most agencies will have a variety of leaflets, brochures, and booklets available. The nurse should check to see what is available. If none seems best for the individual patient, posters and loose-leaf booklets can be easily constructed. Patients with visual problems need large print and/or simple diagrams. Patients with hearing problems need more printed than verbal instructions. Patients with language difficulties will profit from simple diagrams. If films or videotapes are used, plans must be made for their showing and the follow-up discussions. Nurses and nursing students are often quite creative in constructing their own visual aids.

The following illustrates the choice of different teaching adjuncts based on assessment of the individual patient. Four patients are hospitalized with cholelithiasis (gallstones). This is a common diagnosis, and the patient education department has a file of material available, including booklets, a videotape, and programmed instruction. The nurse selected the following materials.

Patient A is a 46-year-old, well-educated female with a basic understanding of cholelithiasis. The nurse chose the videotape for use. This was introduced briefly and followed by a discussion between the patient and nurse.

Patient B is a 38-year-old RN who has not been active for 10 years. She is alert and not experiencing acute pain. After completing the assessment and talking with the patient, the nurse chose the programmed instruction, which the patient enjoyed. This was followed by questions and answers.

Patient C is a 62-year-old woman with a sixth-grade education and limited vocabulary. The nurse selected a very basic booklet and went through it page by page with the patient, reading the script and carefully explaining each diagram. The booklet was left with the patient, and the nurse checked later to answer any questions.

Patient D is a 54-year-old man with limited vision. The nurse enlarged the diagrams in the booklet, used large print to convey the basic related facts, and put together a loose-leaf notebook. This was given to the patient and discussed in detail.

Plan of Presentation

Content Outline	Method	Adjuncts
Brief outline of points to be covered If more than one nursing diagnosis included in plan, note diagnosis to which the content applicable with A, B, etc.	Note method to be used with various items in outline	List specific materials collected or prepared
	Keep notations parallel with content outline to indicate method and adjunct to be used with different areas of content	

Table 8.4: Plan of presentation.

Implementation/Evaluation

The implementation of the teaching plan simply follows the outline. This link is central in patient teaching. If well planned, there should be few problems. The plan may cover several sessions. If so, it should be in a format that other members of the nursing team can follow, since the same nurse may not be able to complete all sessions.

Time

After assembling the teaching materials, a definite time must be established if not previously done. The patient should be allowed some input regarding the time preferred. Hours after morning care and doctor visits are a good time for many patients, who may be tired by afternoon. Others will prefer afternoon hours following a brief rest after lunch. Some who have few visitors may prefer evening hours to fill the time. If the family is to be included in the teaching, this must be considered. Some of the family may spend most of the day with the patient, or a phone call may be necessary to have a member come in. After setting the time, it is essential that the nurse make certain that responsibilities for other patients will not interfere with the teaching session.

Many teaching sessions will be short, 10 to 20 minutes. This is especially true if the patient has received written material ahead of time. A large part of the session will be assuring that the material was understood. If a skill is involved, numerous short sessions are better than a few long ones. For example, if the patient needs to learn how to give an injection, the first session is best limited to withdrawing the solution from a bottle. The time allowed and number of sessions will depend on the content to be taught as well as the individual patient.

Setting
Some arrangements may need to be made for the setting. If the patient is in a private room, there are no problems. A semiprivate room is not necessarily a hindrance, since some roommates would be interested and enjoy the teaching. Whatever location is selected must be acceptable to the patient.

Patient Participation
Patient participation reflects the success of the teaching plan, since effective teaching involves both participants in the teaching/learning situation. The plan may need further adaptation after starting. If the patient seems bored, the nurse should switch to a different approach. If the patient appears tired, the plan can easily be changed to a greater number of shorter sessions. The nurse must be flexible in teaching as in any nursing care.

Evaluation
Evaluation should be ongoing during the teaching process and when the teaching is completed. It is the link that determines whether the previous links should be replaced. The evaluation of learning should relate to the goals that were mutually set. Properly worded goals help establish factors to be included in evaluation. They clarify what is to be evaluated and often include how the evaluation is to be accomplished. Unless the learner responds in some form, the teacher is unable to fulfill the responsibility of evaluation.

Evaluation may be accomplished in several ways. The patient may be requested to respond in a verbal form, a written form, or a psychomotor form. Cognitive learning may be evaluated in an oral, written, or application form. The nurse may ask the patient to state facts that have been included in the content, to write the answers to a list of questions, or to apply the knowledge to a situation such as selecting foods for a diet that was the topic of the teaching. Any psychomotor skills must be evaluated by the patient's performance.

Affective learning requires ingenuity in evaluation. Determination of adherence to a prescribed regimen may be considered evidence of the patient's acceptance of the condition. Observance of behavior when routines are performed can give clues to the patient's feelings regarding a pathological condition. For example, when teaching a patient to irrigate a colostomy, refusal to look at the stoma indicates nonacceptance of the colostomy. This obstacle is difficult to overcome but not impossible. It may require a change of approach such as irrigations by the nurse for a few days with no attempt to make the patient perform the procedure. As the nurse exhibits an accepting attitude toward colostomy irrigation, the patient may tend to be more accepting and gradually participate in the procedure.

Self-monitoring is sometimes used as a method of evaluation. This is not readily adaptable to short-term use. It is more effective in the area of behavioral changes such as regimens for weight reduction. The patient must be self-motivated to make the change and be willing to keep behavioral records for self-monitoring to be effective.

All evaluation does not take place after the teaching is completed. In college courses, what would be the reaction of students to having only a final examination in each course? Learners need to be appraised of their progress during the learning period. Both knowledge and skills should be evaluated periodically, many times immediately. This is especially true of skills. The longer a person is allowed to perform incorrectly, the more difficult it is to change the performance. During the first practice of a skill, any errors should be noted to allow the learner to correct the mistakes. Periodic feedback summarizes the strengths and weaknesses of learning at intervals and serves to increase long-term retention.

Evaluation should be in a form that enhances self-esteem and motivates the patient to continue the learning process. Any successes should be praised and any difficulties minimized. If the nurse is certain that the answer is known, the patient may be asked to explain a facet of the illness to a family or friend. This increases self-esteem as the new knowledge is displayed.

After evaluating the patient's learning, it may be necessary to completely revise the teaching plan and begin again. Before starting over, the nurse should carefully evaluate the approach. What factors seemed to interfere with the learning? What teaching strategy might appeal to this patient more than the one used? Was it the patient's physical or emotional condition that blocked teaching? There must be a reevaluation of items in the assessment, approaches used, any barriers to teaching/learning, and a determination of possible changes that could make the plan more effective.

Implementation/Evaluation

Time	Setting	Patient Participation	Evaluation
Date and Time May be more than one session	Where Individual or group Environment Support persons present	Verbal/written/behavioral response Spontaneous remarks of patient/support person Any return demonstrations	Evaluation method used Patient/support person's achievement Was the goal met? Is follow-up needed? Would another method be more effective?

Table 8.5: Implementation/evaluation.

Documentation

All teaching/learning sessions must be documented in the patient's record. This serves multiple purposes, such as: communication to other health team members, proof of fulfillment of teaching requirements as specified by accreditation agencies and the nurses' job description, and a legal record of the teaching provided and patient/family response.

Careful documentation can prevent or win lawsuits. Problems may arise after a patient is discharged. If there is documentation of the fact that teaching was provided and the patient and/or family evidenced understanding, the nurse will not be held liable for any charges that might be brought related to patient education.

The purposes of documentation indicate some of the information that should be included. There must be a notation of the general subject matter included in the teaching. It is important for the patient/family response to the material presented to be recorded. Achievements should be in specific terms. If, for example, a patient's daughter has been taught to give insulin injections, the documentation should reflect the fact, as in Figure 8.3.

9/22	0930	Insulin procedure demonstrated to patient and daughter, Corinne. Patient refuses to attempt self-injection at this time. *L. Norman, RN*
	1300	Patient's daughter, Corinne, demonstrated ability to withdraw solution into syringe. *L. Norman, RN*
9/23	1030	Daughter, Corinne, accurately demonstrated injection procedure using orange. *L. Norman, RN*
9/24	0730	Daughter, Corinne, demonstrated ability to perform insulin injection by preparing and giving insulin to patient. *L. Norman, RN*
9/25	0730	Insulin correctly administered to patient by daughter, Corinne, without assistance. *L. Norman, RN*

Figure 8.3: Documentation of patient teaching.

There would be intervening entries in the documentation in Figure 8.3, but this is an example of documenting patient teaching. It shows that the procedure was taught and that it was correctly demonstrated by the daughter more than one time prior to discharge. The notes reflect the fact that the patient did not want to give the injections. It clearly documents patient education regarding insulin injection and is legal evidence that would support the nurse's claim to having adequately taught the procedure.

Sometimes there are subtle or not so subtle cues that the patient does not understand or will not follow the information presented. These observations should be recorded without any of the nurses' opinions. For example, a cardiac patient was instructed about a program of rest and activity with specific exercises to be gradually increased over a period of time. The following was documented.

Accurately planned prescribed exercise routine for the first week following discharge. Stated, "I don't have time for all of that stuff. Besides, it sounds boring, I'll just do it whenever I can."

This shows that the teaching was done and the patient understood it, but it does not imply adherence.

Documentation is the last link in the chain that forms the patient teaching process. The evaluation may have indicated a break in the chain that required a return to the planning and implementation. Documentation should reflect this break. The process may start all over as additional learning needs are identified.

These may or may not be related to the original problem, but it is the responsibility of the nurse to follow-through on any identified learning needs.

STANDARD TEACHING PLANS

Nurses are generally familiar with standard nursing care plans, which are excellent guidelines. Nurses who are new to the profession or new to an institution will find them invaluable. They specify routine care the agency expects the nurse to deliver. Standard teaching care plans serve the same purposes. The teaching plans are usually developed within the health care setting and include points that meet the agency's teaching standards. Like nursing care plans, they specify guidelines but must be adapted to the individual patient.

Standard nursing care plans should include at least one nursing diagnosis related to patient teaching. Patient teaching is part of overall nursing care and not a separate entity. Frequently the learning needs will be identified on the care plans with goals and interventions included. Other institutions have separate teaching plans that are linked to the care plans and considered supplementary to care plans.

Standardized teaching plans are definitely timesavers and excellent if used properly. They are not developed as a tool to be used with every patient but as guides to patient teaching. The plans are developed for a particular illness or pathological dysfunction. They include the general items of information and skills that are usually required for care following discharge from the hospital.

As an example, a portion of a standard teaching plan is noted in Table 8.6. This would serve as an excellent plan for many patients, but Mr. Taylor was an exception. He was not convinced that he had a heart attack and was resistant to following any instructions. His wife spent a lot of time with him and seemed genuinely concerned about his attitude. Martha Sims, his nurse, decided that enlisting the cooperation of Mrs. Taylor was essential in reaching Mr. Taylor. She talked with Mrs. Taylor privately.

Content	Method	Teaching Aids	Evaluation
Myocardial Infarction			
Pathophysiology	Discussion	Pamphlet	Recall/discussion
Contributing factors)			
)	Discussion	Videotape	Question/answer
Signs and symptoms)			
)			
///			
Other Treatments			
Diet	Discussion by dietitian	Diet booklet	Menu selection
Exercise	Discussion	Pamphlet	Program plan for after discharge

Table 8.6: Excerpts from standard teaching plan.

Instead of trying to explain the pathophysiology of a heart attack or showing a videotape, Martha made a poster listing signs and symptoms of myocardial infarction. She went over this briefly with Mr. and Mrs. Taylor and left it in the room. This gave the two of them a chance to discuss it and gave Mr. Taylor time to think about his condition. Hopefully, he would realize that he had suffered a heart attack.

Martha talked casually with the patient and his wife several times during the next 2 days about his signs and symptoms prior to admission. Mr. Taylor came to the realization that he had suffered a heart attack. Martha then utilized the videotape suggested in the teaching plan and was able to follow-through on the remainder of the plan with Mr. Taylor's full cooperation. Had Martha tried to apply the standard teaching plan without adapting it to the situation, the teaching would have fallen on deaf ears.

Mrs. Washington, who was also hospitalized following her second heart attack, was another exception. The chart from her previous hospitalization noted that patient teaching had covered the information included in the standard teaching plan. Through questioning, Martha determined that Mrs. Washington understood the teaching but was not complying with the doctor's recommendations. She was still 50 pounds overweight and refused to follow an exercise program. Martha decided to use a contract teaching approach and concentrate on diet and exercise. The dietitian was contacted to again discuss the diet program. Martha talked with the doctor regarding follow-up after discharge. Both were very supportive of her plan. She modified a teaching contract to include a chart for the patient to record daily dietary intake and exercise. Martha included Mrs. Washington in formulating the goals and the chart so that it would require the least amount of time and effort. Through team efforts, the patient was convinced of the seriousness of her condition and the need for following the regimen.

Standard teaching plans would be the perfect answer to patient teaching if all patients fit into the same mold. However, since patients are individuals with differing needs and abilities, these plans must be adapted. Standard teaching plans serve to save nurses time in formulating plans for the routine items to be included and leave them time to be creative in developing goals and interventions to meet individual patient needs.

CHECK IT OUT

Obtain a standardized teaching plan from your clinical facility that would be applicable for a patient who has been assigned to your care. Consider how well it could be used with your patient by answering the following questions.

Was the plan appropriate for the developmental level of your patient?

Were any teaching aids included or suggested?

Could you have used it with minimal if any adjustments?

Can you suggest a different approach for teaching the same material?

APPLICATION IN THE CLINICAL SETTING

Various facets in the teaching/learning process have been discussed, as well as some approaches in application. The next step is to apply this knowledge in the clinical situation by preparing and implementing a teaching plan. The suggested format that has been introduced in this chapter is a guide that may be used in writing a teaching plan. As with the nursing process, a longer form is presented to the student than will be used after becoming familiar with all of the steps.

Figure 8.4 is an example of a completed teaching plan on the suggested format. Notations of pertinent information to be included in each section have been presented in this chapter with a discussion of each part. Completing this form may seem time-consuming at first, but much of the information will have been obtained from the patient assessment for planning care. This is another link between patient teaching and the care plan. Learning needs are identified in conjunction with all physical and emotional needs of the patient, making teaching an integral part of overall patient care.

Patient assessment

Factors Affecting Ability to Communicate	Learning Readiness	Sensory Status	Learning Needs
Alert 68-year-old female Retired school teacher Basic understanding of medical terminology	Not acutely ill Concerned about infection from minor wound left leg Experiencing some pain at intervals	Wears glasses Hears normal tones Some limitation of motion of left hand	Knowledge of sterile technique Wound irrigation and dressing change procedure Knowledge of measures to prevent wound infection

Nursing Diagnoses	Goals

A. Knowledge deficit: Wound irrigation and dressing change procedure	A. Demonstrate wound irrigation and dressing change correctly before discharge
	   1. Recall basic principles of sterile technique as presented in videotape
	   2. Demonstrate wound irritation
	   3. Demonstrate dressing change

B. Self-care deficit: Prevention wound infection	B. Demonstrate understanding of prevention of wound infection by:
	   1. Recall signs & symptoms of wound infection
	   2. State methods of preventing wound infection

Figure 8.4: Patient teaching plan.

Planning considerations

Resources Needed	Available/ Arrangements	Patient's Support System	Nurse's Support System
Private room	In private room	Daughter visits daily	Standard teaching plan adaptation
Videotape dressing change	Schedule use	Arrange time with her	Approved by physician and head nurse
Irrigation and dressing supplies	Available on unit		
Booklet on wound care	From Pt. Ed. Dept.		
Specific irrigation instructions	Write instructions with diagrams		

(Page 2) Plan of presentation

Content Outline	Method	Teaching Aids
A. Dressing change	A.	A.
1. Basic principles of sterile technique	1. Discussion	1. Videotape
2. Wound irrigation	2. Demonstration	2. Prepared instructions with diagrams
3. Dressing change	3. Discussion demonstration	3. Videotape
B. Prevention wound infection	B.	B.
1. Signs and symptoms wound infection	1. Oral presentation	1. Booklet
2. Preventive wound care	2. Discussion	2. Booklet

Implementation/evaluation

Time	Setting	Patient Participation	Evaluation
10/4 1000	Conference room	Watched videotape with interest, verified concepts following	Verbally noted basic principles presented
1400	Patient room	Recalled details from videotape. Observed, then completed irrigation with daughter's assistance	Basic concepts correctly stated. Accurately demonstrated irrigation procedure
10/5 1000	Patient room	Irrigated wound and changed dressing with daughter's help. Recalled signs/symptoms wound infection and proper wound care	Demonstration accurate. Correct recall wound care. Goals are met No follow-up needed

Figure 8.4 cont'd.: Patient teaching plan.

Documentation

Date/Time	Nursing Progress Notes
10/4 1000	Patient and daughter viewed videotape on sterile dressing changed. Expressed interest.
1400	Recalled basic concepts of sterile technique. Demonstrated correct wound irrigation technique with daughter's assistance, followed demostration by nurse.
10/5 1000	Daughter assisted in wound irrigation and dressing change. Procedure correctly completed. Recalled symptoms of wound infection and wound care.

Figure 8.4 cont'd.: Patient teaching plan.

Patient teaching is a legal responsibility of the nurse, but it is also a very personally rewarding activity. Patients often express appreciation for the nurse's taking time to help them understand their condition in terms that are meaningful to them. But it should be kept in mind that patients often have a lot that they can teach the nurse. When assessing patients' basic knowledge regarding their current illness, the nurse should try to determine the knowledge patients may have to share. They may have read widely and talked with specialists about a specific diagnosis and treatment or have firsthand knowledge of the use of an appliance. A patient with an artificial larynx may be eager to demonstrate its use.

Patients can make the material in textbooks come alive if the nurse just takes the time to listen. As students put knowledge to use in patient teaching, they should keep in mind that some authorities feel that skill in teaching is the result of practice. Thus it is important to practice at each and every opportunity. In making preparations to teach, the teacher often learns as much as the student. The nursing student or practicing nurse as well as the patient will benefit from patient education.

IN A CAPSULE

The *teaching process* follows the format of the nursing process with the specified addition of documentation as a last step. An *educationally focused assessment* includes factors affecting ability to communicate, learning readiness, sensory status, and learning needs. The *nursing diagnosis* indicates the specific area of the learning need. *Goal setting* should involve both participants who formulate mutually acceptable, realistic, measurable goals that are patient centered within an established time frame. *Planning* must consider the available resources and support systems as well as the selection of content, strategy and adjuncts best suited to the content chosen.

The *implementation* of the plan takes place at an opportune time and is adapted to the individual patient. *Evaluation* may be in verbal, written, or psychomotor form at intervals during the teaching and at the end of the teaching/learning process.

Documentation of patient/family teaching should specify the learner response as well as the material taught. *Standard teaching plans* are time-savers and excellent guidelines to be adapted to the individual patient.

DO YOU REMEMBER

- the steps in the teaching process?
- factors affecting the ability to communicate?
- areas to be assessed in determining learning readiness?
- the effect of sensory status on teaching/learning?
- nursing diagnoses related to teaching/learning?
- various details to be considered in planning teaching?
- what should be included in the documentation of teaching?
- how standard teaching plans can be used effectively?

CAN YOU DESCRIBE

- specific assessments of learning needs?
- the approach to goal setting and the components of a well-written goal?
- the implementation and evaluation phase of the teaching process?

ACTION, PLEASE

1. You have been assigned to prepare a teaching plan for a 62-year-old man with a third-grade education who needs to learn to cleanse and change dressings on a leg wound. Plan the approach you would use from the following selections.

Teaching Strategy
A. Role play
B. Discussion
C. Demonstration
D. Lecture

Adjuncts
A. Videotape
B. Model
C. Prepared booklet
D. Handmade posters

You may combine more than one strategy and use more than one adjunct to teaching. Give your rationale for each choice. Briefly describe the general approach you would use.

_____

_____

_____

_____

_____

_____

_____

2. *How Would You Document This?* Cheryl Lyons is a high school student who was involved in an automobile accident. She has a fractured mandible with her teeth wired together. You have attempted to teach her to take fluids through a straw, to suction, and to perform oral care. Cheryl has been very uncooperative and makes only halfhearted attempts to care for herself even though she is scheduled to go home tomorrow. You have called Mrs. Lyons to ask her to come to the hospital for you to explain the procedures, but she said she doesn't have time.

a. How would you document the teaching?

_____

_____

_____

b. What would you specify regarding Cheryl's response to teaching?

_____

_____

c. Would you document contacting Mrs. Lyons? If yes, how would you word it?

_____

_____

d. Would this documentation protect you legally?

_____

_____

UNIT II BIBLIOGRAPHY

Bille, Donald A. *Practical Approaches to Patient Teaching*, Boston: Little, Brown and Company, 1981.

Cross, K. Patricia. *Adults as Learners.* San Francisco: Jossey-Bass Publishers, 1982.

Cunningham, Margaret A. and Baker, Dennis. How to Teach Parents Better and Faster. *RN*, September, 1986.

Ellis, Janice R. and Nowlis, Elizabeth A. *Nursing: A Human Needs Approach.* Boston: Houghton Mifflin Company, 1985.

Falvo, Donna R. *Effective Patient Education: A Guide to Increased Compliance.* Rockfille, Maryland: Aspen Systems Corporation, 1985.

Kozier, Barbara and Erb, Glenora. *Fundamentals of Nursing: Concepts and Procedures*, Third Edition. Menlo Park, California: Addison-Wesley Publishing Company, 1987.

Megenity, Jean S. and Megenity, Jack. *Patient Teaching: Theories, Techniques and Strategies*. Bowie, Maryland: Robert J. Brady Company, 1982.

Miller, Ann. When Is the Time Ripe for Teaching? *American Journal of Nursing*, July, 1985.

Picariello, Gloria. A Guide for Teaching Elders. *Geriatric Nursing*, January/February, 1986.

Rankin, Sally H. and Duffy, Karen L. 15 Problems in Patient Education and Their Solutions. *Nursing 84*, April.

Rankin, Sally H. and Duffy, Karen L. *Patient Education: Issues, Principles, and Guidelines*. Philadelphia: J. B. Lippincott Company, 1983.

Smith, Carole E. Patient Teaching: It's the Law. *Nursing 87*, July.

Taylor, Judy A. Are You Missing What Your Patients Can Teach You? *RN*, June, 1984.

Taylor, Rosemarie A. Making the Most of Your Patient Teaching Time. *RN*, December, 1987.

Trekas, Joanne. It Takes 2 to Achieve Compliance. *Nursing 84*, September.

Woldum, Karyl M., et al. *Patient Education: Foundations of Practice*. Rockville, Maryland: Aspen Systems Corporation, 1985.

Nurses' Communication With Health Care Personnel

9

Nurses' Communication Within the Health Care Organization

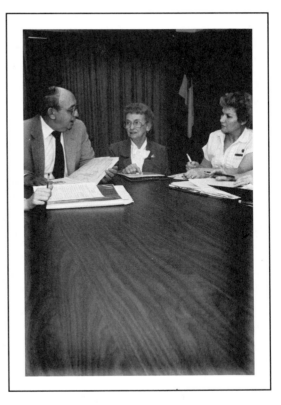

Life is not so short but that there is always time for courtesy.
Ralph W. Emerson

OBJECTIVES

Upon completion of this chapter, the student will be able to:

- describe communication within the hierarchy of an organization.
- note the role of the nurse as patient advocate.
- note the importance of observing the proper channels of communication.
- state the impact of attitude and timing on communication.
- explain the concept of territoriality in the health care setting.
- list considerations in telephone communication.
- note variances in group structure.
- state the influence members may have within a group.
- compare the effects of cohesion and conflict within a group.

- describe behaviors and influences that facilitate or hinder the group process.
- differentiate styles of group leadership.
- discuss interactions within a student group.
- compare assertive, nonassertive, and aggressive behaviors.
- state the significance of assertive communication in the workplace.
- note the effects of conflict within an organization.

GLOSSARY OF TERMS*

Aggressiveness   Tendency toward dominating or mastering another.

Assertiveness   Ability to confidently declare convictions in a positive manner without infringing on rights of others.

Autocratic   Characterized by authority in one person.

Cohesiveness   Exhibiting a closeness or sticking together.

Democratic   Relating to active participation by all members with decisions made by a majority.

Laissez faire   Characterized by lack of direction in actions.

Territoriality   Persistent attachment to a specific territory.

*Definitions applicable to content.

This unit focuses on communication within the health care setting but is not centered on direct communication with patients. The topics discussed do, however, have a bearing on patient care. Communication with health care personnel affects the general atmosphere of the facility. It directly influences approaches to patient care through shift reports and patient conferences. The nurses' notes reflect care given to patients and serve as communication with health care team members. Communication with other health care personnel has an effect on nurses' job satisfaction, which is reflected in patient care.

This chapter is concerned with communication in the health care facility. Organizational structure and common-sense hints on communication etiquette are included, as well as a discussion of small group interactions.

GENERAL ORGANIZATIONAL COMMUNICATION

Interdependency

There is interdependency within any organization. In order for a facility to function effectively, the people must work together harmoniously and be aware that every position is important. An example of this is the janitor in an organization who saw the job as one of the most important because no one could function in an atmosphere of dirty floors and overflowing trash. Only when individuals in the health care facility see their roles as indispensable will the organization operate smoothly. The job satisfaction of employees is affected by a mutual feeling of interdependency.

It is obvious that health care facilities would not remain open if doctors did not admit patients. The doctors must realize that their patients would not receive adequate care without the efforts of the entire hospital staff. Administrators must realize that the hospital cannot function without nurses. Nurses must be aware that even the lowest staff position is an essential cog in the wheel. All ancillary department personnel must realize that their contributions are absolutely necessary for the welfare of the patient.

Formal and Informal Rules

Rules are necessary in any organization to keep things running smoothly. Some rules are written, formal policies. New employees are often given a handbook with organizational charts and standard procedures for everything from reporting on duty to requesting a transfer. These remain fairly stable with personnel notified of any change. There are also invisible rules, the "way things are done here." These may be difficult to discover. Only by observation and appropriate questioning can these rules be determined.

Although informal rules change more often than formal ones, no one is notified of these changes. Following a vacation a nurse might return to the same unit to find the nurses charting in a different location, the medication room rearranged, or the division of duties altered. These rules or norms are not carved in stone, but the staff adheres to them. The staff member who has "seniority" on the unit may consider it a prerogative to initiate or approve any changes. Many rules are created to save time or to complete tasks more efficiently. The existing group maintains those norms they consider most acceptable but resists change, especially changes suggested by a newcomer.

There are formal and informal rules that apply to channels of communication in an organization. The informal norms allow for short-circuiting as a means of saving time or correcting errors. However, this will result in a personal debt, as shown in the following situation. Paula was an RN on a medical unit. Her friend Alice was a lab technician. Paula had forgotten to order a fasting blood sugar, so she called her friend.

> *Paula:* Alice, can you please come up right away and draw a blood sugar.
> *Alice:* I was just up there 15 minutes ago and didn't see the requisition.
> *Paula:* I know. I forgot it.
> *Alice:* OK. I'll do it this time.

This was fine, but Paula was now in debt to Alice, and the opportunity to collect wasn't long in appearing. Alice was now in a bind.

> *Alice:* Paula, I know the late trays have already been brought up, but can you hold Mr. Halton's tray. I dropped his blood sample and must get another.
> *Paula:* But his food will get cold.
> *Alice:* You owe me one. Remember the blood sugar last week?

So Paula sidetracked the tray until the blood could be drawn, then had to warm it before serving.

This is a very minor situation and easily resolved. However, favors and shortcuts can lead to major personal problems and to legal problems in some instances. For example, if a supervisor should be notified under certain circumstances, a short cut cannot be used. The proper channels must be followed in making the report because this transfers part of the responsibility to the supervisor.

One of the most difficult things for a nurse who is new in an organization to learn can be the informal rules. Any questions may be interpreted as insecurity on the part of the new nurse. But how else can one learn aspects of the job such as who is responsible for scheduling, how to requisition supplies, to whom an injury is reported, or which doctors strongly object to being called at night? Questions should never reflect need of reassurance or apology for having to ask. For a person to be accepted and feel part of any organization, questioning is a necessary part of self-orientation.

Acting as Patient Advocate

Communication within the organization may involve the nurse in the role of patient advocate. Some health care systems have an ombudsman or patient advocate on the staff. This person may or may not be a nurse. If there is no such position, the nurse can work in this role. Patient advocacy should be the responsibility of all health care professionals. Unfortunately, however, this does not always hold true.

It is sometimes suggested that the advocate can work to change the system by revealing any injustices and inadequacies. The patient advocate can see that the system does not prevent the delivery of what the patient should rightfully expect. This aspect presents concerns. The physician or hospital administrator may believe that a nurse is overstepping the role in acting as patient advocate when carried to this point. If the nurse reports unethical or illegal behavior, will this raise a question of employment being jeopardized? Who will support the nurse who conscientiously acts as patient advocate? Nursing needs a support system for conflict in the employment situation regarding implementation of the code of ethics. Fortunately, most health care facilities support the nurse who presents adequate evidence of unethical behavior.

COMMUNICATION ETIQUETTE

Nurses interact with numerous persons within the health care setting. There is a certain amount of protocol observed in any institution, from schools to churches to political settings. There are also rules of the game in communication within health care settings. Communication etiquette in the health care setting is similar to that in any business relationship. Problems arise when established protocol is not observed. Problems are usually compounded when stress levels are high. This factor emphasizes the importance of observing the rules in health care environments, in which interactions often occur in the midst of stress.

Channels of Communication

Observing the proper channels of communication is important in all communication. For example, if a person buys an item from a local chain store and is dissatisfied, the president of the corporation would not be contacted. The first action would be to return the merchandise to the local store. If satisfaction is not received, further steps could then be taken. Personnel can create problems by not following channels of communication within the framework of an organization. Communication channels follow the hierarchy of authority. Therefore, it is wise in any new situation to become familiar with the organizational structure, whether it is a school, business organization, hospital, or any other institution.

For a student in a nursing program, any problem in the clinical area should first be discussed with the clinical instructor. If the problem deals with classroom teaching or testing, the specific instructor should be the initial contact. If employed in a hospital setting, the head nurse on the unit is the first person to contact. This is not to say that the initial contact is the end of the line. If unable to solve the problem after contacting the first person in the chain of command, the next level of authority should be made aware of the circumstances. Every institution has an organizational chart showing the lines of authority, and most college handbooks have a stated grievance procedure. Regardless of the institution or situation, the levels of authority should be followed until satisfaction is obtained.

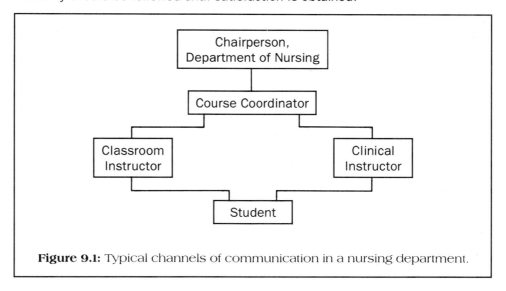

Figure 9.1: Typical channels of communication in a nursing department.

Problems are magnified when channels of communication are ignored. Complaints may be brushed aside if a person complains to a higher authority in the organizational hierarchy. It may preclude obtaining a fair audience at a later date if the complaint is not initiated at the proper level. The problem is inevitably referred back to the proper channel, and the person involved will be aware of the fact that they were not consulted first. When properly approached, the average person with authority will listen to reason. Problems can usually be solved without a resultant straining of working relationships.

Attitude

Many problems stem from lack of or miscommunication. With an approach such as, "I may have misunderstood what you said. . .," or "Can you please clarify. . .," most problems can be resolved. On the other hand, confronting an instructor with comments such as, "Why do I have to do all this work when Mike didn't?" or "My paper was as good as Mary's but you didn't accept mine," is almost certain to cause a problem between the student and instructor.

Verbal Encounters

The person initiating communication sets the tone for the interaction. The attitude with which a person is approached can be a deciding factor between a satisfactory solution to a problem and continuing frustration. A hostile approach puts the other person on the defensive, creating an instant block to any meaningful communication. If anger results in anger, then it follows that a friendly approach will result in the same response. For example, the head nurse makes out the schedules on the floor where Eloise was hired to work with the understanding that she would be off every other weekend. When the following month's schedule was posted, Eloise noted that she had only one weekend off, so she stormed into the head nurse's office.

> *Eloise:* You plainly told me that I would only have to work every other weekend. Now you have me scheduled for three weekends next month. I don't think you're fair. You let the people you like off and schedule me to work.
> *Head Nurse (in an icy tone):* The schedule will stand as it is posted.

Is the head nurse's response typical? How should Eloise have approached the head nurse? It must be remembered that everyone can make mistakes. The head nurse could have made an error in the scheduling and might have corrected it if Eloise had inquired in an acceptable manner. Only with a positive approach can an atmosphere conducive to open communication be created for the exchange of ideas necessary to reach a mutually satisfactory solution.

Nonverbal Indicators

Body language projects an attitude that may be more convincing than words. The manner in which something is said, the posture, the gait, and the facial expressions may imply a friendly or hostile attitude. However, a subservient attitude should not be used in approaching a superior when there is a problem. An open, honest approach to the discussion of an area of concern is appropriate.

Timing

Timing is an essential factor in establishing a positive atmosphere for communication. This factor, which was discussed in relation to nurse-patient communication, also holds true in other situations. An effective communication interaction requires the readiness of both participants. This cannot occur if one person is involved in a conversation or activity that is demanding attention. No one welcomes interruptions when involved in a project that requires concentration. A time that is more appropriate should be chosen.

When someone initiates communication, there is a reason. This places communication in the realm of goal-directed communication. This can be more effective if an appointment is made. A block of time is then reserved to discuss the situation.

This is only common courtesy. When accompanied by respect, this yields productive communication.

Territoriality

Territoriality in Physical Space

Territoriality is sometimes considered synonymous with or closely akin to personal space. Personal space relates more to how close another individual stands or sits next to a person, while territory involves areas, objects, or activities claimed as one's own. It is a well-known fact that members of the animal kingdom establish a boundary of the territory they wish to inhabit. This functions as a protection against overcrowding through proper spacing. Humans tend to establish a territory but for other reasons. Everyone tends to have a favorite place, a special chair at home, or a preferred seat in class. Some people place personal articles in a place to mark their territory. Patients in hospitals or residents in nursing homes establish a territory, which provides a sense of identity or a feeling of control. This is true even though the space may be extremely limited.

Territoriality in Responsibilities

The concept of territoriality extends beyond the bounds of physical space in the work situation. It deals with behaviors used to manage or defend one's area and the responsibilities or privileges considered to be private property. It is the areas a person considers to be off-limits to others in the realms of decision making or functions performed. It is seldom in writing or communicated to newcomers but can be a source of misunderstanding between people, as illustrated in the following situation.

> Robert was new on the oncology unit but was familiar with the procedures. On his second day he noticed that Mr. Pack was having difficulty feeding himself. Since Robert's assigned patients did not need him at the time, he helped Mr. Pack with his breakfast. At noon Robert sat down at the table with Martha, who worked on the same unit. She turned away and refused to talk to him. Robert later learned from another nurse that Martha considered Mr. Pack her special patient and always requested to care for him whenever he was admitted. She resented Robert's invasion of her territory.

Had Robert spoken to Martha before assisting Mr. Pack, a misunderstanding would have been avoided.

The concept of territoriality can be considered a part of communication etiquette in that knowledge of co-workers' territory must be determined and respected. Just as it is an intrusion of privacy to demand attention from others when they are obviously busy, so it is an invasion of their territory to assume duties designated "theirs" without asking permission.

Management of one's territory involves seeking help when necessary as well as protection of boundaries. The territory an individual can manage is related to size, skills, and experience. To function effectively and maintain good working relationships, another person's responsibilities should never be assumed uninvited. Instead, willingness to help when asked will result in a better work situation.

Telephone Etiquette

Telephone communication is a part of interactions in health care settings. The faceless voice at the end of the phone line can convey efficiency in taking doctor's orders, empathy in answering an inquiry about a loved one, or a cold uncaring attitude. The manner in which the phone is answered gives the caller a general impression of the institution. The nurse is a representative of the health care facility, whether talking on the phone or talking directly to patients and visitors.

The same rules of telephone courtesy apply as in business—identification of location and person speaking, a pleasant tone of voice, and a willingness to listen to the caller and to give the information requested or to connect the caller with the proper person. Unit secretaries answer the phone initially in most hospitals, but the amount of information they are allowed to dispense or receive is limited. The nurse usually has the responsibility to conduct any phone communication with doctors, to receive reports, and to talk with families.

Telephone conversations cannot be supplemented with nonverbal components; therefore, messages must be carefully encoded to minimize misunderstandings. The factors that make a verbal message more effective—simplicity, brevity, clarity, relevancy, and credibility—are even more important in phone conversations. Verbal clarification of messages is essential in the absence of the nonverbal component.

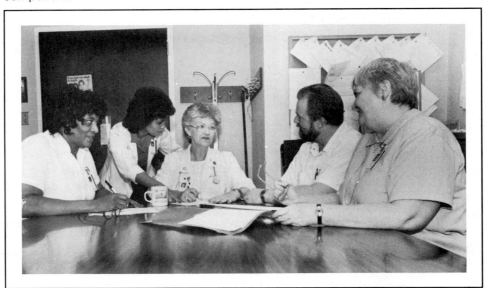

SMALL GROUP INTERACTIONS

People in general function within different groups in many ways. The family is the first basic group into which a person is incorporated. Preschool and school are next for a child. Adults function in numerous groups, such as social groups, church groups, volunteer community groups, and political groups. Nurses are involved in many different types of groups formed for many different purposes. The composition of the groups varies from those composed entirely of nurses to groups with other health care professionals or families of patients. The groups may be formed to solve problems, to coordinate efforts, or to make future plans. The groups may be small or large, directly or indirectly concerned with patient care, or professional nurse groups. To function most effectively within any group, an understanding of different types of groups and their structures and procedures is essential.

Group Structure

Group Size

Groups will vary in size according to their general purpose. Large groups can exert influence but have a disadvantage in that it is next to impossible to reach a consensus of opinion. Any large group functions with smaller committees, in which most of the work is accomplished. Small groups allow for more active participation by each member. However, if these groups are too small, they may not provide enough different viewpoints or ideas. Interaction of group members and satisfaction with the outcome of the activities of the group are greater in relatively small groups. The ideal group size is one that is large enough to accomplish the goals but small enough to allow each individual to participate actively. The following discussion deals primarily with small groups.

Membership

The membership in some groups is relatively stable. This facilitates accomplishment of the purpose of the group. When there is a frequent change within the membership, time must be taken periodically to update new members on the progress of the group. Members may be assigned to some groups, with or without an expressed preference, while the membership of other groups consists of volunteers. Those members who choose to be a part of the group usually tend to be more committed than those who are assigned.

Meetings

Finding a meeting place and a time acceptable to all members of a group may be a problem. The meeting place would probably not be a particular problem for a small group but could be very difficult if the group was very large. In small groups, the preference of each individual is considered in selecting a time. However, this is impossible with a large group. Frequency of meetings is another consideration. If meetings are scheduled at frequent intervals, members may complain of the time required to serve in the group. If the meetings are too far apart, members often lose interest.

Group Process

Group process, like nursing process, involves collecting data, defining the problem, establishing a goal, planning, carrying out actions necessary to achieve the goal, and evaluating results. Interpersonal communication skills of the group members play a big part in the functioning of the group. Aspects of group process to be considered include the approach to discussion, rules of the group, influences within the group, and behaviors that facilitate or hinder the group process.

Approach to Discussion

Groups utilize discussion to work toward establishing a goal and planning activities to reach this goal. Informal discussion is used in daily living as people discuss schoolwork, child rearing, gardening, or vocations. Group discussion is more formal in that it is aimed toward meeting a goal or solving a problem. Group discussion may consist of free encounters but should be disciplined. The discussion must stay on the subject in order for the task at hand to be accomplished.

In the group process people share ideas with others. Large corporations sometimes have meetings called "think tanks" or "brainstorming" sessions in which ideas, regardless of how implausible they sound, are bounced about in an attempt to reach a new approach to solving a problem. No idea is criticized until all members have had an opportunity to present possible solutions. This approach is appropriate in a defined problem area in which there is no obvious answer to the problem. It is less useful when applied to a broad problem area. These sessions should be planned when time is not a critical factor, because brainstorming cannot be rushed if it is to be successful. An effective group incorporates this concept by encouraging each member to express any ideas for consideration in working toward a productive end.

CHECK IT OUT

Try brainstorming with a small group, or call it a think tank if you prefer. Choose one of the problems below or use an actual problem area in which you are involved. Listen to all that each person has to say regardless of how farfetched the idea sounds. Let the ideas flow freely and see what innovative plans you can devise.

1. Interest in the student nurse association has been very low. How can you get more students involved?
2. Class morale is at a low ebb due to generally low grades on the last two tests. How would you approach this problem?
3. The nurses on each shift on the unit are complaining about their workload being heavier than that of the other shifts. What would be the starting point in resolving this?

Group Rules

Some groups adhere to very formal rules for the conduct of business, such as those found in *Robert's Rules of Order*. Other groups have less formal and often unstated sets of rules. Members learn the unwritten rules as they work within the group. Consistent negative responses or behaviors that interrupt group discussion should be disallowed by an unwritten rule in any group. Most groups have other unwritten rules that are consistent with common courtesy, such as never interrupting the speaker. Active participation may be mandatory in a group. This requirement can be very productive but may cause some individuals who do not like to express their ideas to avoid the group.

Influences within the Group

Often when a group of people are working together, one or more individuals will seek to influence the direction of the work and the outcome of any decisions made. There may be a clique within a group that attempts to influence others, and they may be able to direct the course of action followed by the group. In some groups, a person is appointed to serve as chairman for the group. However, in the absence of an appointed leader, persons who are assertive and decisive in action take the lead. This is advantageous only if that person is able to facilitate group action toward accomplishment of the goal. Coercive power may move the group toward the goal at the expense of alienating members. Further goals set for the group are then useless if the members cannot wholeheartedly participate.

Members may influence others in the group in subtle ways, such as rewarding certain behaviors and ignoring others. For example, if one person tends to talk at length on any topic that is introduced, other group members may forego the rule of not interrupting and break into the discourse. If a rather shy person who seldom speaks up starts to relate ideas on a subject, others may actively listen and comment positively on the ideas expressed.

Behaviors that Facilitate Group Process

The effective group member or leader is a good follower. To be a good follower does not mean to follow blindly and do as instructed at all times. It means participating actively in the group, making suggestions when pertinent, and completing any outside tasks. The good follower cooperates wholeheartedly in all activities of the group and accepts decisions made by the majority.

The ideal group member is one who makes every effort to help the group reach the goal by making brief and candid contributions to the discussions. The ability to make oneself understood and to try to understand others is essential to good interpersonal communication and to effective group functioning. The ideal member is friendly and outgoing, actively encourages other members to participate, and strives to maintain group harmony. This person seeks to identify problems and keep the group focused on the goal.

The effective group member completes any outside research assigned and brings the information to the group. This individual willingly accepts responsibility for tasks needed to accomplish the goal and gives suggestions without demanding that they be followed. If all members were within this category, problems would be easily solved.

Behaviors that Hinder Group Process

Unfortunately all group members do not fit the preceding description. Some exhibit behaviors that tend to block progress toward decision making or attainment of a goal. Some individuals in the group may believe that it is a waste of time to fully discuss a problem and demand an immediate decision. Others become very aggressive and are ready to fight to get a suggestion accepted unanimously by the group. Then there are those who deride any idea presented by others but offer no alternatives. These members are the nonconformists, in that they oppose any idea that is presented, as shown in the following example.

> Lenore was a nonconformist. She was a member of a group that was formed to plan in-service staff education programs. The following excerpts from a meeting typify Lenore's participation.

> *Carol:* I think a presentation on lithotripsy would be of interest.
> *Lenore:* No one wants to hear any more about that stuff.
> *Harold:* I would suggest a review of body mechanics since we have had six nurses off with back strains.
> *Lenore:* We did that 2 or 3 years ago and it didn't do any good.
> *Marion:* We really need to present the new chart forms.
> *Lenore:* That's silly. Everyone can read and figure them out.

> Anything accomplished by this group was in spite of, instead of with Lenore's help.

Some members tend to block all action by the group. They believe that the entire group is irresponsible and that any action taken would prove to be dangerous. The goal or tasks of the group have no meaning for them. Others may become members only for the recognition and because the committee membership looks good on their record. They constantly stray away from the current group discussion to talk of their pet projects. There are numerous other subtle ways in which one or two members of a group can hinder the group process, such as refusing to make any contributions to discussion or refusing to let others talk. Some always agree with whatever is said. The latter may be a group reaction when a prominent member of the group expresses an opinion. All agree during the meeting but later express dissatisfaction. A look at these negative aspects may be helpful in seeing what not to do.

Comparison of Behaviors in Group Interaction

Facilitative Behaviors	Behaviors that Hinder
Friendly and outgoing	May become aggressive
Seeks to identify problem	Believes group is irresponsible
Makes brief, candid suggestions	Wants suggestions accepted or offers no opinion
Keeps focused on goal	Strays away from topic
Tries to understand ideas of others	Derides ideas of others but offers no alternatives
Encourages others to participate	Will not let others talk
Strives to maintain harmony	Demands immediate action

Table 9.1: Small group interactions.

Group Leadership

The behaviors considered have been those of members of a group. But what about the leader? The chairman of a group may be appointed or may assume the role if, for example, committees are on a rotating basis and the member having served the greatest length of time becomes chairman. Some leaders are selected by the group when it is first formed. Regardless of the method of selection of a leader, that person does not always exhibit leadership qualities. The most effective leader may be the one who emerges as the members work together. Each leader will adopt a slightly different approach to leadership, but the leadership styles can be loosely categorized as autocratic, laissez-faire, or democratic. It always holds true, however, that the good leader is also a good follower.

Autocratic Leadership

This type of leadership is also called authoritarian. The person considers it a great honor to have been chosen to lead the group and feels a sense of responsibility. The autocratic leader decides what the group should do and attempts to induce members to act accordingly. Tasks may be assigned to members and their ideas discussed, but the final decision will be made by the leader. Autocratic leadership is sometimes said to be efficient in that is less time-consuming than other approaches. However, time should not be the only consideration. Members find little satisfaction from participation in the group when their contributions are never seriously considered. They are not committed to supporting decisions in which they have had little or no part in reaching.

Laissez-faire Leadership

In this situation the leader exerts little influence on the group, the leadership role may rotate, or there may never be a specific leader, little is accomplished. Some group participants may see the situation as nonthreatening and enjoy the relaxed atmosphere. Others may view their participation as a waste of time. Groups with this style of leadership need a goal and a purposeful focus. If a strong leader does emerge, the group may either become a productive entity or be led away from the intended purpose.

Democratic Leadership

A democratic atmosphere is by far the best approach to group leadership. The democratic leader helps the group identify problems, set definite goals, and work toward accomplishing them. Individual members are encouraged to participate in discussions. Innovative ideas are welcomed, and the entire group discusses possibilities of trying a new approach to solve a problem or develop a program. The leader may change periodically as members volunteer or are selected to lead the discussion of a topic in their field of expertise or interest.

The democratic leader provides a general direction for the group but also encourages each member to share responsibility for the activities and accomplishments of the group. Decisions are made following discussion within the group and reached through a consensus of opinion. The decision may not be unanimous, but the leader assists the members in reaching a compromise. Members in groups with democratic leadership are committed to any decisions made and the leader works *with* the group in all activities.

CHECK IT OUT

Make a list of several small groups in which you have particpated in the past year or so. The group interests need not be limited to health care, but strictly social groups should not be used. Apply the following questions to each group.

1. What specific actions of members seemed most helpful in moving the group toward its goal?
2. What behaviors, if any, impeded the progress of the group?
3. What type of leadership was exhibited by the chairman?
4. How effective was the group in terms of meeting the goal in the amount of time allotted to do so?

Review the process and accomplishments of each group to determine factors that contributed to their productivity.

Rate yourself as a group member on a scale of 1 to 10, with 10 being the ideal group member.

Student Groups

A discussion of small groups would not be complete without some mention of student groups. While the preceding information is applicable to student groups, there are some special considerations. The discussion is more applicable to the clinical group than the classroom situation, which is different in general structure. Clinical groups usually work closely together in caring for patients over a period of time and develop relatively close relationships. The group interaction extends from conferences that take place before the clinical work and clarify assignments for the day to postconferences that follow the clinical time.

Postconferences are a time for learning, for sharing experiences, and for gaining insights from classmates. Students are encouraged to share their experiences of the day. Any problems that have arisen can be discussed in the group. The problem might be one of communicating with a patient or one encountered in bedside care of the patient. It might be feelings that arise in caring for a dying patient. There may be a problem between the student and a staff member. Some student-staff problems can be aired in the group, but some should be discussed only between student and instructor. Most problems can be resolved when faced directly.

Students are expected to actively participate in postconferences. Instructors often assign students on a rotating basis to lead discussion. These discussions are usually related to the current area of study and designed to reinforce classroom learning. The serious student will spend time in preparing a presentation. As noted in patient teaching, the teacher, or leader in this case, learns in preparing to teach. This is another situation in which the student can share what has been learned with classmates.

People can be the type of group member they choose to be. This applies to the nursing team, which actively cares for patients, to students, who participate in clinical conferences, and to members in any group. The manner in which people decide to lead the group is their choice, as is the type of group member they choose to be.

RELATIONSHIPS WITHIN THE ORGANIZATION

The nurse is constantly interacting with individuals in the health care setting. General organizational communication with rules and etiquette that should be observed as well as interaction in small groups have been discussed. There are some additional specific reactions of individuals that have an effect on relationships within groups and within the organization that should be considered.

Assertiveness in the Workplace

Assertiveness is the ability to declare convictions openly and honestly. It is the sharing of thoughts and emotions in a positive manner with confidence. Assertive people make their own decisions and stand up for their convictions. The assertive person is empathic in trying to understand others and listens without interruption to what others have to say. Assertiveness is usually linked with strength and capability. Assertive people tend to be sure enough of themselves to be able to freely reveal feelings.

Expressing Assertiveness

To say that a person is assertive does not indicate that all feelings in every situation will be revealed. There are times when even the most assertive person will be hesitant to speak out. For instance, if a superior issues a directive that there will be

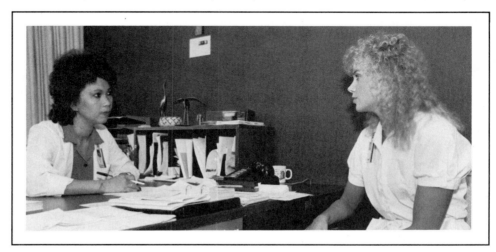

a change, it is foolish to try to object if it is a minor matter that does not involve patient safety or job security. The assertive person neither expresses nor suppresses all feelings. To verbally express every felt emotion would border on the abnormal, while suppressing all emotions gives life a sterile quality. The ideal is the use of discipline in sharing feelings in a present situation without bottling emotions up for a torrential outpouring at some later date.

Assertiveness Involves Choice

Everyone has a choice in all situations. People are not compelled to act in a particular manner. Choice is an important factor in being an assertive person. Assertive people do not allow themselves to be manipulated by others or by circumstances. The realization that choices are available and that it is not necessary to accept dictates of another if these happen to be against personal convictions is a comforting thought. The assertive person will speak out to defend convictions.

Nonassertiveness

Nonassertive people are the opposite. They consider themselves inferior and always agree with others. These individuals have difficulty in expressing feelings. They stay in the middle of a bad situation because they do not want to do anything to offend anyone.

Nonassertive individuals allow others to make decisions for them, letting others direct the course of their lives. They stay in the background and verbally agree with whatever is said. These people avoid making decisions by putting things off, thinking they do not have to accept responsibility if they have not voiced an opinion in any decisions made. They tend to think of themselves as being less capable than others and are not completely happy.

Assertive versus Nonassertive Responses

The following example compares typical assertive and nonassertive responses in a situation.

> Mr. Belford, the hospital administrator, visited the weekly head nurses' meeting, at which the main topic of discussion was shift scheduling. Mary and Beth were both at the meeting. They were good friends, and were both very efficient head nurses with high staff morale on their units. They had previously discussed the issue and both agreed on the many advantages of flexible staff scheduling that had been in effect for the past year. Mary was an assertive person, and Beth was the opposite. The following responses illustrate the differences.

> *Mr. B.:* There has been some dissatisfaction expressed with the flexible scheduling we have been using. I think it is time to return to a uniform scheduling policy on all units with all nurses working 6 days followed by 2 days off, which gives an occasional 4-day weekend. I would like your opinion on this.

> *Beth:* It should work out if you think it will. I'll be more than happy to make out next month's schedule on that basis.

Mary: Mr. Belford, I have tried the scheduling you are recommending and it does have some advantages. But the nurses on my unit have been much happier with the flexible scheduling approach as they are better able to correlate their work and family responsibilities. The unit is adequately covered at all times, and the nurses have repeatedly expressed their satisfaction in having some choice in their work schedule.

Even though Beth liked the flexible scheduling, she was unable to stand up to Mr. Belford and state her convictions. Mary, an assertive person, is able to accomplish things, while Beth, a nonassertive person, is strictly a blind follower who can be led in any direction.

Aggressiveness

Assertiveness is not the same as aggressiveness. Aggressive people try to impose their position on others, to make decisions for other people. They consider themselves strong and capable and constantly try to manipulate others. These are the people who interrupt in a loud voice to call attention to themselves. Because they consider themselves more capable, they find fault in others to make themselves look better. They have no regard for the feelings of others but are concerned only in having their own way.

Assertiveness in Action

The assertive person contributes to progress in working toward a goal within a group or within an organization. The aggressive member tends to block effective interactions and creates an atmosphere of tension. The nonassertive individual does not make any waves but offers few suggestions and rarely questions any decisions made. The assertive persons listens to others but makes decisions based on what the individual considers right. This person tries to understand positions taken by others and shows a willingness to talk through any problems. Assertive people communicate openly and honestly with others. This encourages a fuller expression from others. Assertive people accomplish things.

Becoming More Assertive

From looking at the contributions made by assertive, nonassertive, and aggressive people, it seems obvious that assertiveness is to be desired. Anyone can become more assertive. One of the first steps is to take responsibility for all actions. People can control their own behaviors. If they allow others to judge what they do, then they are being manipulated. To be assertive, one should not apologize needlessly. There are times when an apology is in order, but people may try to manipulate others by demanding explanations. Everyone should observe common courtesy and apologize briefly when indicated, but not for every action.

Assertive people are not afraid to change their minds. Making mistakes is in the same category. Everyone learns through mistakes. If an error in judgment is made, the mistake should be admitted. Assertive people do not feel that everyone has to like them, because this leaves the door open for manipulation. Nor is it necessary to have a burning interest in everything. It should always be possible to express lack of interest. The assertive person should feel free to make requests of others as well as to refuse requests that are made of them.

Assertive people are those who are able to accomplish changes and are comfortable with themselves. Assertiveness may cause a degree of conflict for a short period but will open the door for productive discussion, compromise, and progress toward achieving any goal.

Conflict and Cohesion in the Workplace

Groups exhibit conflict and cohesion in varying degrees. Conflict is inevitable in any organization, just as in groups. Conflict occurs when differences meet and ideas are in opposition. Conflict does not have to be destructive. The manner in which it is handled is the key to the outcome of conflict.

Causes of Conflict

Conflict may stem from communication breakdowns when messages are not decoded as sent. Prejudices may be a factor in the manner in which people react to others and disagree with them without cause. People may jump to conclusions without stopping to learn all of the details of a situation. Sometimes personnel within an organization oppose any new ideas or actions without considering the possible benefits of the change. Communication skills and a large amount of patience are needed to deal with these situations.

Resolving Conflicts

Conflicts must be resolved as soon as possible for working conditions to be acceptable. It is essential to get as much information as possible to start in the right direction in resolving a conflict. In obtaining the information, several answers to the problem usually come to light. The information obtained must be sorted out and organized. Any conflict has numerous ramifications, because it is never simple. Both sides in the conflict must try to take an objective look at the opposition.

To cope with conflict, the nurse should acknowledge its existence and allow the other person to verbalize differences. It is best to try to find the basic cause rather than the incident that triggered the confrontation. A conflict cannot be resolved until it is pinpointed and the events leading up to it identified. This can help to avoid future conflicts.

Conflict may arise from a personal attack of one person by another. Prejudices or biases may be the basis of a conflict situation. The responsibility for these situations may rest primarily with one individual. Personal counseling followed by open communication between the parties involved with a neutral person present may be effective in resolving the conflict.

Conflict arising from a power struggle may be a serious problem. Any power struggle is detrimental to progress and to working relationships. There must be open communication and cooperation between the individuals involved if the conflict is to be resolved.

Any conflict is a two-way street, not the problem of only one individual. There does not have to be a winner and a loser, because both parties can be winners if the situation is handled well. They need to work together to attempt to understand the other person's viewpoint and determine the direction to proceed. Any conflict is reduced with understanding.

Positive Effects of Conflict

Conflict does not necessarily have only negative effects. It may be preferable to apathy resulting from lack of interest. In working in groups, conflict can indicate that members are committed to the problem and have independently tried to find solutions. The presentation of differing ideas as possible solutions to the problem may create a conflict. However, by considering all suggestions, an answer to the problem may be found as the conflict is resolved.

Confronting issues and constructively resolving conflicts can actually improve group relationships. Behaviors of the members of the group influence the manner in which conflict can be dealt with and resolved. It can have a positive outcome if viewed as a means of progress in interpersonal relationships. It may be seen as a means of adjusting self-image, of responding to a perceived threat to status, or of assertion of what individuals consider their rights. It can indicate interest in and commitment to a problem. If conflict is met in a straightforward manner and people involved are able to compromise on issues, all viewpoints can be fully explored and a satisfactory result achieved.

The first step in resolving a conflict is to define the point of difference and events leading up to the current situation. Each person should be allowed to express an opinion or state a position. Clarifying messages by asking if the message was understood as intended can be crucial in resolving a conflict. Conflicts do not have to be a win-lose situation. Solutions can be reached that are acceptable to all parties concerned. There is always a satisfactory answer to any conflict, although finding the right compromise may take a little time.

Cohesion

Cohesion is defined as the process of sticking together. Cohesion within a small group or within the workplace results when there is agreement on the goals and everyone works cooperatively to achieve them. The commitment of the personnel results in a feeling of accomplishment on the part of the individuals.

The cohesive group strives to keep the group process going, to maintain a viable entity that identifies problems and solves them. These groups are the ones that recognize surmountable obstacles and are able to overcome them. Any disagreement within the group is resolved by the members. Through creative thinking, the group finds innovative solutions to problems.

Health care facilities are ideally cohesive organizations with all personnel working toward the goal of more effective patient care. This is more difficult to attain in large institutions than in smaller ones, but it is not impossible. Open communication between all personnel is essential. Extreme cohesiveness, however, is said to have a somewhat stifling effect since everyone agrees with each suggestion and few new ideas surface. This is not seen often enough to be considered a problem.

IN A CAPSULE

For *communication within an organization* to be effective, the interdependency of departments must be acknowledged and rules observed. One aspect of the nurse's communication within the organization may relate to *patient advocacy*.

Communication etiquette in the health care setting involves following the proper *channels*, a positive *attitude*, attention to *timing*, and respect for others' *territory*. Since the nonverbal component is missing, *telephone communication* must be carefully encoded and statements clarified.

Group structure varies according to the size and purpose of the group. Any *group discussion* should be open with each member encouraged to present ideas. *Group rules* should be followed whether these rules are formal or informal.

Members within a group may attempt to *influence* others in subtle or in coercive ways. The ideal group member takes responsibility for tasks and promotes participation by all members, which enhances an atmosphere of harmony that *facilitates group process*.

The *group process is hindered* by members who oppose all ideas presented, who agree with all that is said, who never offer suggestions, or who push to have all of their proposals accepted. The *group leadership* style may be *autocratic* or *laissez-faire*, but the *democratic* approach is usually most effective. An example of small group interactions applicable to *student groups* is the postconference meetings of clinical groups.

Assertive persons contribute to progress and are able to accomplish change by stating their convictions. They are willing to listen to ideas of others and make compromises. *Nonassertive* people contribute little toward progress or change because they seldom offer an opinion. *Aggressive* individuals disrupt interactions and hinder progress.

Some *conflict* within an organization can lead to progress and better working relationships if personnel are willing to compromise in resolving an issue, but is detrimental if triggered by a power struggle. *Cohesion* within an organization, if not in the extreme, fosters accomplishment.

DO YOU REMEMBER

- what is meant by interdependency in an organization?
- how the nurse can act as patient advocate within the organizational framework?
- the impact attitude and timing can have when initiating communication?
- how the concept of territoriality can affect working relationships?
- the basic rules of telephone courtesy?
- the manner in which one or more members can influence the group process?

- the types of group leadership?
- the interactions of students in clinical groups?
- the positive and negative effects of conflict and cohesion?

CAN YOU DESCRIBE

- overall communication within an organization?
- problems that arise when the proper channels of communication are not followed?
- variations in group structure?
- critical factors in small group discussion?
- the positive and negative effects of cohesiveness and conflict within a group?
- behaviors that facilitate group process?
- disruptive behaviors of group members?
- behaviors exhibited by assertive, nonassertive, and aggressive personnel in the workplace?

ACTION, PLEASE

1. Obtain an organizational chart of your school and clinical facility. Place names in the positions if known. In both school and clinical situations, trace the channel of communication from you to the head of the organization.

    a. You received a "D" in a nursing course, but you think you should have gotten a "C" according to the grades you had received during the semester. If you aren't satisfied with the response of the first person you talk to, what would you do?

_____

_____

_____

    b. You are a staff nurse and have received a written reprimand for a medication error, which was actually made by another nurse. What recourse do you have?

_____

_____

_____

2. How would you perform as a group leader?

You have been working on a medical unit for 6 months. The head nurse assigns a staff nurse to lead a discussion on a condition or procedure that may be unfamiliar or not well understood by the staff. The nurse assigned to lead the discussion is allowed to develop the session in any manner comfortable. Co-workers may be asked to present specific aspects of the discussion.

You have been in enough discussion sessions to observe the behaviors of the staff members. Grace attempts to dominate any discussion, Jim usually offers positive comments, Paul tries to impress others by recounting unrelated personal experiences, Harriet never enters into the discussion, and Charlotte and Sarah are quiet but always cooperative.

    a. Which co-workers would you ask prior to the meeting to present areas of information? Give rationale.

_____

_____

_____

    b. What ground rules, if any, would you make at the beginning of the discussion?

_____

_____

_____

    c. What would be your style of leadership?

_____

    d. How would you respond to Grace if she started on a lengthy discourse?

_____

_____

_____

    e. If Paul strayed from the subject to relate a fantastic rescue he made, how would you handle the situation?

_____

_____

_____

    f. What approach would you use to involve all of the staff in the discussion?

_____

_____

_____

3. *Assertiveness* The patients on the unit on which you are working in a nursing home all need assistance with activities of daily living. The staff is minimal, making it difficult to effectively care for all of the patients. At a staff conference the head nurse suggests bathing patients on alternate days instead of daily. Consider the following responses.

    1. State whether each is assertive, nonassertive, or aggressive.

    2. Note what your response as head nurse would be to each.

    a. That sounds like a good idea. It certainly will give us more time for other aspects of care.

    1. _____

    2. _____

b. That's the silliest thing I ever heard. I manage to take good care of all of my patients. They need a bath every day.

    1. _____

    2. _____

c. That might be a possibility, but I feel that these patients need the daily skin care to prevent decubiti.

    1. _____

    2. _____

10

Nurses' Communication with the Health Care Team

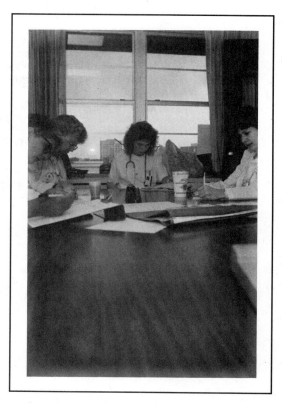

True friendship is like sound health; the value of it is seldom known until it is lost.

Charles C. Colton

OBJECTIVES

Upon completion of this chapter, the student will be able to:

- explain special points in communication between nurse and nurse, subordinate and superior, nurse and aide, student and staff nurse, physician and nurse, and nurse and ancillary department professionals.
- discuss interdisciplinary team communication.
- list purposes of written records in the health care setting.
- note the general information that is included in the patient charts.
- state uses of written memos that are not included in the patient charts.
- discuss legal implications relative to patient charts.
- describe the concept and current sta-

tus of nurse-patient privileged communication.
- list factors to be considered in planning a patient care conference.
- give an effectual shift report on one or more patients.

GLOSSARY OF TERMS*

Ancillary   Supplementary; something that adds to or makes complete.
Interdisciplinary   Involving two or more academic or scientific fields of study.
Litigation   A legal contest carried on through the judicial process.

*Definitions applicable to content.

The previous chapter dealt with communication within the health care setting in general. This discussion will center on face-to-face as well as written communication with the health care team, with the exception of nurses' notes, which will be covered in the next chapter. Effective communication with the health care team promotes congenial working relationships, which indirectly increases the quality of patient care.

FACE-TO-FACE COMMUNICATION WITH HEALTH CARE PERSONNEL

Nurses are members of the health care team. As such, communication with other members of this team is imperative. Interactions involve peers, superiors, and subordinates, with the aspect of patient welfare superseding all other concerns. There may be times when relationships with other members of the health care team will be strained to the breaking point if their requests or instructions are not considered to be best for the patient. This is the time to be assertive in playing the role of patient advocate.

Nurse/Nurse Communication

Peer Relationships
Communication with other nurses that is directly related to patient care on a health care unit is on a peer level, even though one nurse may be considered superior to the other in title and area of functioning. These relationships must be mutually supportive for the unit in the health care facility to operate smoothly and patients to receive optimum care. Self-concept has an influence on the manner in which people communicate. A high self-concept makes people "feel good" about themselves. Nurses usually are concerned about helping others to feel good, but there should be some consideration of self. When individuals accept themselves as worthwhile, they are able to help others to attain this same sense of self.

Communication Approach
Nurses develop a professional identity apart from a personal identity. Some may show this professional side in such a manner that emotions are never expressed, leaving the impression of being unfeeling. The nurse who is able to express

emotions to co-workers tends to develop a closer working relationship. The typical ideals of social service and expertise basic to the nursing profession carry weight in communicating with other nurses and health care personnel. These ideals create a spirit of cooperativeness in working together for quality patient care.

Many items discussed in group interactions are directly applicable to nurse/nurse communication. Assertiveness in communication with other nurses enables each to express ideas regarding approaches to patient care. Care must be taken not to cross the line to aggressiveness and attempt to impose ideas on others.

Subordinate/Superior Communication

Nurses communicate with those above them in authority and with others beneath them in the chain of command. Most communication on this level will be within the nursing department. However, there are occasions when nurses communicate with hospital administration. This may be related to a new program or to equipment needed or may be initiated by administration in response to a complaint.

Communicating with Superiors

One area of communicating with superiors deals with evaluation of performance. This may be a scheduled annual conference or may be the result of a specific incident. When in the subordinate position, the nurse should ascertain the purpose of the meeting beforehand in order to plan and prepare, as shown in the following example.

> You are a staff nurse and have an appointment with the supervisor regarding medication errors that occurred on your shift. You should check on the facts, and if you were directly responsible you should be prepared to take the consequences. If you were not the responsible party, you should have as much information available as possible with specifics on the sequence of events. This is not a matter of informing on a co-worker but a statement of facts. A strong caution in this type of situation is to remain in control of your emotions and avoid any demonstration of anger.

A nurse initiating communication related to a problem in working relationships or scheduling should follow the channels of communication within the organization. There should be no hesitation in carrying a request or grievance to a supervisor if unable to obtain satisfaction at a lower level. Other aspects noted in communication etiquette should be observed in communicating with a superior.

Communicating with Subordinates

The RN communicates with subordinates within the nursing department in day-to-day working relationships. Many of the communication interactions deal with care of patients, since the RN coordinates the duties of LPN's and aides. Most of these relationships tend to be like that of a peer relationship with the patient's interest the primary concern. Some of the relationships involve another RN when one is in a position such as head nurse or supervisor.

One of the most difficult areas for many nurses involves reprimanding a subordinate. It is even more important to remain in control of emotions when in the superior position than in the subordinate one. It is easy to tell others that they are doing a great job, but an annual evaluation can be stressful to both parties concerned if the performance has been less than satisfactory. Any reprimand or appraisal should be face-to-face. To hand a person a written evaluation is the coward's way out and creates distrust and resentment.

When a reprimand is necessary, mention of positive aspects of behavior in the individual along with the performance in question will promote a continued satisfactory working relationship. In criticizing the performance of a subordinate, only statements reporting facts should be used. Any judgmental statements severely hinder further communication, and inferences leave room for misinterpretation. Anything other than straight facts arouses emotional responses and creates ill feelings. Threats of firing should be used only as a last resort.

CHECK IT OUT

Working in pairs, have one person play the part of the head nurse and the other one a relatively new staff nurse. The head nurse reprimands the staff nurse in one of the following situations.

1. The staff nurse has been 15 to 20 minutes late for work the past 3 days.
2. One of the patients assigned to the staff nurse had requested pain medication and did not receive it for about 40 minutes. This occurred during the time the staff nurse had gone to lunch and another nurse was caring for the patient.
3. It was called to the attention of the head nurse that the staff nurse had been very discourteous in refusing to assist a patient to the bathroom on three occasions.

Nurse/Aide Communication

Nurse/Aide Relationship

A nurse/aide relationship is a superior/subordinate situation, but it also applies to everyday general working relationships. Many aides have worked in the health care facility for a number of years, are experienced in their tasks, and do not question the authority of the nurse. However, an aide may be placed in an awkward position when there is a change in the nurse in charge. The nurse may have different priorities and expectations than the nurse with whom the aide previously worked. Sometimes these differences are not communicated to the aide.

Nurse's Responsibility

It is the responsibility of the nurse to let the aide know what is expected and take time to answer any questions. The nurse should tell the aide the reasons for requesting specific activities and information. This establishes a relationship in which each trusts the other and provides an atmosphere of mutual respect.

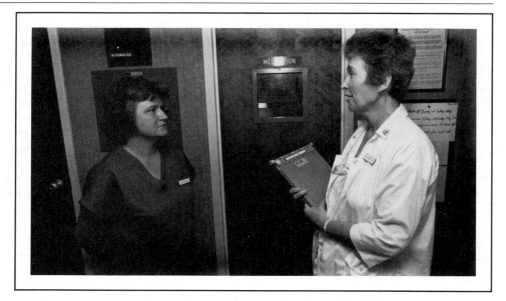

The experienced aide should be relied on to use good judgment in areas within the realm of designated responsibilities. Since aides spend considerable time at the bedside of patients, they can frequently offer creative solutions to problems. Aides should be included in planning care. This increases their feeling of self-worth and adds to a feeling of satisfaction in the job. The nurse who takes the time and opportunity to communicate with the aide can often improve patient care on the unit as well as create a mutually beneficial relationship with the personnel.

Student/Staff Nurse Communication

Students in the clinical setting face communication problems that are different from those of nurses working in the health care facility. They work with the staff nurses but also are responsible to the clinical instructor. The student/staff nurse relationship will vary. The staff nurse may assume a superior position or may keep the interactions on a peer level. Students who are freshmen will be viewed differently by the staff nurse than senior students or experienced nurses who are furthering their education.

Learning Experience

The student is assigned to the clinical facility for a learning experience. The day of an apprenticeship approach to nursing education has disappeared. Instructors should carefully choose experiences for students that are related to current classroom topics and within the student's level in the nursing program.

Students must have time during clinical experience to carefully review charts and to observe procedures by various other health care professionals. They need time to communicate with patients and put into practice the techniques of communication. Students must have time to learn through the numerous activities that contribute to a productive clinical session.

Limit of Student Activity

The nursing staff must be made aware of procedures that can be performed by students, regardless of any experience the student may have had in a clinical facility. The student is held responsible for actions in caring for patients. Nursing activities must be restricted to those procedures that have been presented in the classroom and/or practice lab. If the instructor posts a list of procedures that students are allowed to do, there should be no doubt on the part of students or staff of the student's ability to carry out these procedures.

Student/Staff Relationships

A complementary working relationship can develop with the staff performing in the position of superior and promoting productive experiences for the student. This is the relationship most frequently seen. Most nurses remember their student days in the strange new environment of a health care facility with pressures of time and performance increasing stress levels. They empathize with students, sometimes to the point of trying to protect them.

A positive relationship may not be established between student and staff in all situations. There are a few staff nurses who view students as being in the way and invaders of personal territory, as incapable of performing anything but the basic procedures, or as a personal "gopher." The instructor must intercede for the student in these situations to assure adequate clinical experience.

Nurse/Physician Communication

Nurses frequently complain about doctors, but often very little is done about it. Most complaints are about the older doctor who started practicing when nurses played the role of handmaiden, following orders with never a question and running on the double to fulfill any request. Nurses want to be recognized for their abilities and knowledge.

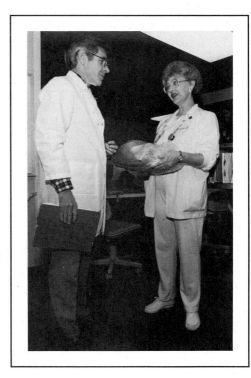

Changing Concepts

The concept of the nurse in the inferior role to the doctor has undergone many changes in the past few decades. As nursing has moved toward a professional level with more stress on education, there has developed a blurring of functions in some areas. The emergence of the nurse practitioner has led the nurse to expect more equality with the physician. The nurse has assumed additional responsibilities but does not want to usurp the physician's role.

Physicians may react negatively toward nurses because they feel threatened that nurses will move into medical practice. This is not what nurses want. Their educational background does not prepare them to be diagnosticians, but it does prepare them to assess patient needs and work toward meeting them. It might be said that the physician works toward diagnosing and treating pathological conditions while the nurse's role is that of diagnosing and treating human needs.

Differentiation of Roles

The fact remains that doctors are cure oriented while nurses are care oriented. The adoption of the term "nursing diagnosis" has caused concern for many of the older physicians who have not been able to see the difference between a nursing and a medical diagnosis. The medical diagnosis speaks to the cure aspect, the nursing diagnosis to the care aspect.

Some nurses feel awed and threatened by physicians. They fear being reported to administration if an order is questioned or if a task within the realm of nursing is performed without a specific order. Open communication between nurses and physicians is the only way to close the gap between the two.

Communication Approaches

A "doctor/nurse game" is sometimes seen in which there is no winner. The game is usually a subtle one. Any suggestions by the nurse must be hidden so that the physician can claim the idea. The nurse may assume the submissive role on the surface, which avoids any penalties such as being labeled aggressive. The nurse obliquely suggests what the doctor should do. The doctor assumes the responsibility but does not directly accept the nurse's suggestion, which would be acknowledging the expertise of the nurse. This can be a comfortable game for many, but it fails to acknowledge nurses' status in the health care team.

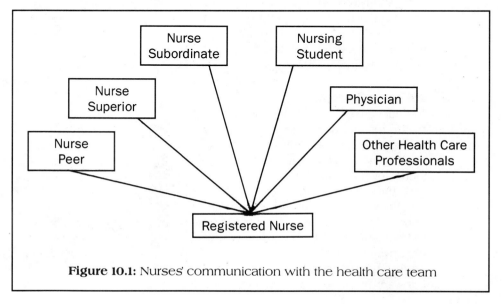

Figure 10.1: Nurses' communication with the health care team

If the nurse is to be an effective communicator, skills must be applied in communicating with physicians in an open manner. Honesty in letting the physician know if there is disagreement on a point of patient care is essential. Physicians may listen to nurses they consider competent. Assertiveness in establishing a working relationship as partners in providing quality care for all patients is the ultimate goal of nurse-physician communication.

Nurse/Ancillary Department Professionals Communication

The nurses' relationships with professionals in ancillary departments in the health care facility are considered peer relationships. Each has an area of expertise and should work cooperatively for maximum benefit to the patient. Communication should provide feedback and clarification of goals. There may be some difficulty related to approaches in organizing health care, but each professional can learn from the other. It is well worth the nurse's time to listen actively to the other professionals and to establish mutual respect in the relationship, from which the patient is the prime benefactor.

Interdisciplinary Health Team Communication

Cooperative Approach

Some health care facilities are placing more emphasis on an interdisciplinary approach to patient care. Representatives from the various departments that are directly concerned with patient care are consulted regarding their area of expertise. In some institutions, the team will make rounds together and discuss patient needs. The team often includes physician, nurse, dietitian, clinical pharmacologist, and dentist plus other specialties that may be indicated such as speech therapist, physical therapist, occupational therapist, respiratory therapist, social worker, or psychologist.

Cooperation among the team members significantly increases the quality of care the patient receives. When there is open communication, each team member is able to make a contribution in planning care and in scheduling activities for effective care without tiring the patient with tight scheduling. A team approach assures better continuity of care and more efficient management of interdependent problems.

Team Interactions

Many questions will need to be answered in these team meetings to secure maximum participation in the best interest of the patient. Who will be the primary patient communicator? Who will coordinate the scheduling of any treatments or activities? Communication among the interdisciplinary team members may be hampered by different terminology used by various members. Each member should feel free to clarify any language not fully understood.

To look at the overall picture, each member of the team is essential. The doctor may order physical therapy for a patient. The effectiveness of the therapy is enhanced by the therapist's ability and knowledge of the current status of the patient. The nurse further increases the effectiveness of the therapy by reinforcing the therapist's instructions and having the patient prepared for the therapy sessions. Only through the efforts of the entire team will the patient receive maximum benefits.

Many aspects of communication in the health care setting have been considered. The approaches and specific communication techniques discussed in Unit I, Nurse-Patient Communication, are applicable in all circumstances. The effective communicator is able to apply the facilitative techniques in any situation to keep channels of communication open and avoid misunderstandings. It is much less time-consuming to clarify messages immediately than to try to straighten out misunderstandings at a later date.

WRITTEN COMMUNICATION WITH THE HEALTH CARE TEAM

Written communication is an integral aspect of patient care because it is not possible to remember all of the information regarding the patients for whom the nurse is responsible. Written records allow the health care team to obtain the necessary information for quality patient care at their own pace and within the time frame of their schedule. Written communication contributes to accuracy and serves as a later reference.

The written record should also reduce the number of times a patient is required to give the same information. Unfortunately, this is not always true. Health care personnel may repeatedly ask for information that is recorded on the patient's chart. This could be avoided if all health care professionals would read the patient's chart and accept the assessments of co-workers. The written record does have some disadvantages in that it may be misunderstood. Ideally, although not always possible, written communication is supplemented by verbal messages.

Purposes of Written Records

Some of the general purposes of written patient records are indicated in the preceding paragraphs. There are specific purposes for written records including communication, education, research, statistics, monitoring quality of patient care, and legal documentation.

Communication

Communication is the primary and most obvious purpose of written records. The written record establishes a data base for further assessments. The nursing team as well as the ancillary departments require written records for the sake of accuracy and avoidance of errors. Medication records, for example, avoid inadvertently repeating the administration of a dosage. Even though verbal reports are given at the end of each shift, the written record allows referral to the patient's general condition and specifics in treatments. Reports from other departments can be checked and physician's orders verified through written records.

Education

Written records are invaluable as an educational tool for students in all health care professions. Nursing students should carefully read the patient's chart before planning care. The chart enables the caregiver to determine the approach that has been used in care, specifics of the patient's current condition, and the history of the illness. It would be very difficult to effectively care for any patient without this basis of information.

Research and Statistics

Patient charts are used extensively for research and statistics. From the data on charts, the effectiveness of various medications and treatments for specific pathological conditions can be studied to determine those that might be most advantageous for current or future treatment of a similar dysfunction. The number of patients diagnosed with specific disease entities, age of patients admitted, length of hospital stay, and seasonal fluctuations aid in planning future hospital expansions and/or structural reorganizations. As more records are maintained on computers, the information will be more readily accessible for research and statistical purposes.

Monitoring Quality of Patient Care

Written records are the primary method of monitoring quality of care. Some audits are performed by outside agencies for purposes such as accreditation and narcotic administration. Nursing audits are routinely performed in many hospitals, with a committee or a permanent staff position delegated to perform the task. The person auditing the records may or may not be a nurse. Standards of care are available to judge the quality of care given. Internal monitoring of quality of care serves to encourage all personnel to maintain high standards.

Legal Documentation

Charts serve as legal documentation and are admissible in court. If patients object to the admission of the record as invasion of privacy, portions of the chart may not be admitted in some instances. Refusal to admit the chart as evidence is usually done only if the data would adversely affect the patient's condition. Legal aspects were noted in relation to patient teaching and will be discussed in more detail later in this chapter.

General Information on Patient Charts

The form of patient charts varies with each institution, but the information on the charts is basically the same. There is always a place for physician's orders and a method for the nurses to record their notation of the orders. The physician's history and progress notes and the records of treatments by ancillary departments form a portion of the permanent record. All reports of laboratory, X-ray, and pathology examinations plus any surgery or anesthesia reports are included in the patient's chart.

Nurses record admission and discharge assessments as well as daily assessments of the patient's condition. Vital signs are recorded on a graphic sheet for easy comparison of stability or fluctuation. Medication records are an essential part of the chart, even though the form will vary considerably. Flow sheets are often used by the nurse for recording routine nursing care to reduce the amount of paper work necessary.

Various records such as preoperative checklists and consent for treatment forms are normally the responsibility of the nurse, even though the physician is responsible for instructing the patient regarding any invasive procedures. Nurses' notes are an important part of the patient record, since they show daily treatments and changes in the patient's condition. The documentation of nursing care is considered in detail in Chapter 11.

Referrals and consultations are not a standard part of patient charts but are incorporated into the permanent record when applicable. Patients may be referred to an outpatient clinic following discharge, for example. This should be part of the record. The primary physician may request the services of one or more specialists. These consultation records are then incorporated in the chart.

CHECK IT OUT

Go through the chart of an assigned patient. Write down in the order noted the categories of information included in the chart. Compare your findings with that obtained by classmates assigned to different clinical facilities.

How did the categories of information on the charts compare?
What differences were noted in the general format?

Written Memos

As noted, written communication is vital to effective patient care. A written and signed record pinpoints responsibility, protecting the conscientious personnel and noting areas of deficiency in those who might tend to be careless. There are many written memos used to enhance effective patient care, even though these memos are not a part of the patient's permanent record.

Interdepartmental Memos

Requisitions to the laboratory, X-ray department, and physical, respiratory, or occupational therapy are a part of interdepartmental communication. These requisitions are recorded within the department and the treatments or reports incorporated in the patient chart. Dietary requests including special patient preferences increase patient satisfaction as well as nutritional requirements. Requisitions for equipment and supplies are necessary to keep any unit functioning. Memos to the housekeeping or maintenance department and even to the employees who rent and/or maintain televisions in the patient rooms are part of the communication within the health care facility.

Nursing Team Memos

Memos are frequently written by nurses to those on another shift. These may be very important for continuity of patient care but may not necessarily be a part of the chart. Nurses may attach a memo to the physician on the front of a chart as a reminder to renew a medication order, to point out a patient request, or to call attention to a change in the patient's condition. Written memos may take the place of verbal communication when it is not feasible, or they may serve to reinforce face-to-face interchanges.

Legal Considerations in Written Communication

Patient charts are legal documents. They are proof of care given. As such, they are used in several ways, such as the audit, to ensure quality of care. Charts are used to confirm all charges made by the accounting department of the hospital when there is any question. Narcotic records are checked by authorities periodically to determine whether all narcotics are accounted for by being charted as administered to patients.

Incident Reports

Any unusual incident or accident should be promptly reported and objective observations accurately documented in the chart. Most hospitals require that an incident and accident report be completed. The physician will usually examine the patient and sign the form. The report is filed in hospital records separately from the chart, but the fact that a report has been completed should not be noted on the chart. This is not an attempt at a cover-up of any sort, since the details are recorded in the nurses' notes. However, inclusion in the chart can have an impact on litigation. If it is not a part of the patient's chart, it is protected by attorney-client privilege and is not admissible as evidence.

Nurses' Notes

Nurses' notes are often checked by lawyers when there is a lawsuit. It is assumed that if something was not charted, it was not done. Some courts take this stance, while others do not. For example, if "AM care" and "PM care" are charted in an institution in which the policy states that these procedures include turning the patient and giving skin care, then it is assumed that the patient was turned and skin care given. The facts, however, must be corroborated by other health care team members. An inclusion in the nurses' notes regarding the skin status of the patient at the time eliminates any question. Nurses are often cleared as a result of their careful documentation of care given and their notation of communication with physicians, supervisors, or family members.

Another area in which the nurse should exercise caution is the consent for treatment form signed by the patient. These forms are not considered valid if the patient does not understand the procedure to be performed or the possible dangers. The nurse should determine that the patient fully understands all ramifications before signing the form. The physician should be requested to explain any areas that are not understood by the patient. Some specifics of nurses' notes with legal implications will be included in Chapter 11.

Litigation

Litigation is becoming more common, with a resultant spiraling of malpractice insurance. All health professionals are held legally responsible in proportion to their level of education, training, and/or experience. This includes student nurses and their instructors. Many lawsuits can be averted or won by accurate and complete charting.

Another aspect to be kept in mind is the fact that patients are more likely to sue professionals they do not like or do not trust. Effective communication tends to decrease the likelihood of a malpractice suit because the patient will trust those nurses with whom there is an open and easy interchange of ideas.

Health care professionals have become keenly aware of the possibility of litigation and should make every effort to avoid it. Some actions to decrease the chance of a malpractice suit include the development of good relationships with all patients, the exercise of due care in charting to protect self, and ascertaining that the patient understands any consent form signed.

PRIVILEGED COMMUNICATION

Responsibility of the Nurse

In the closeness of many nurse-patient relationships, patients share very personal information with nurses. With the privilege of having the confidence of the patient, the nurse has a responsibility to appropriately utilize the information. Facts that may have an impact on the patient's health status should be shared with other health team members when it is the best interest of the patient. Some of this data may be included in the nurses' notes, some may be shared with others in reports or conferences related to patient care, and some may be reported only to the doctor. Other information the nurse may receive will have nothing to do with the health status of the patient and should never be shared with others. It is considered in the realm of privileged information. It is the responsibility of the nurse to determine how to use the information received from the patient, and the decision can be difficult.

There are appropriate places in which nurses can discuss any facets of patient care or communication with the patient. It is inappropriate under any circumstances to discuss these things in public places such as elevators or dining rooms. It is impossible to ascertain whether persons within earshot are in some way acquainted with the person being discussed, even though no names are mentioned. Discussion of patients in public places conveys to anyone who overhears that nurses do not adhere to the concept of privileged communication. Among student groups in conference rooms it is acceptable, but any written information regarding patients should use initials rather than names.

Legal Status

Violating privileged communication is considered an ethical breach of nursing practice that can result in loss of patient confidence. A good nurse-patient relationship depends to a large extent on open communication. This cannot be maintained if the patient suspects in any manner that confidences have been breached. However, the law does not currently protect the nurse-patient relationship with respect to privileged communication in all states. In a recent instance in Utah, the nurse had overheard the patient talking to a lawyer. It was the attorney's client relationship and not that of the nurse that enabled the confidentiality of the patient to be maintained.

COMMUNICATION WITH THE NURSING TEAM
RELATED TO PATIENT CARE

There must be direct communication among members of the nursing team. The information on the chart as well as that contained in the nursing care plans is available to all of the staff, but additional information often needs to be shared to effectively care for patients. Nurses intermittently exchange messages in an informal manner while caring for patients. There are also planned communication sessions with the nursing teams, such as patient care conferences and shift reports, which help to ensure continuity of patient care.

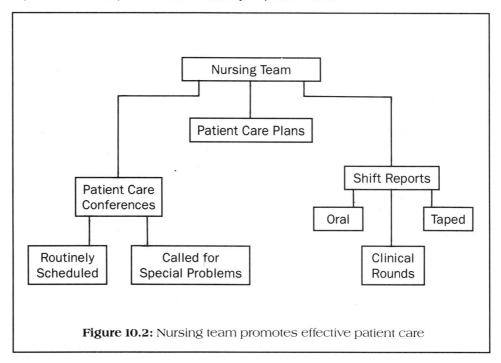

Figure 10.2: Nursing team promotes effective patient care

Patient Care Plans

Nurses communicate with other members of the nursing team through patient care plans. These plans record assessments of unmet needs, selection of nursing diagnoses, plans for nursing interventions or nursing orders, and evaluation of interventions. In some health care agencies, care plans are a part of the permanent record and kept in the patient chart. In others, they are kept in a notebook or Kardex and not filed with the chart.

Nursing care plans are continually evaluated and modified. Responsibility for maintaining current plans varies with the health care facility. The primary nurse is often the person who updates plans and assures their implementation. The responsibility may be on a rotating basis when team nursing is utilized. The mechanics of nursing care plans will not be covered. This is mentioned as only one of the means of communication among members of the nursing team.

Patient Care Conferences

The approach to conducting patient care conferences varies in different health care facilities. There may be several methods used within a single agency. In some institutions patient care conferences are planned weekly or more often, with the staff submitting the names of patients whose care they would like to discuss.

Sometimes a conference is called whenever there is a problem. These may be called by any member of the nursing team or may be requested by a family member. A staff member from another department may be asked to attend any of these conferences if involved in the problem. In other situations there are informal mini-conferences on patient care at the time of shift report.

Arranging the Conference

The person designated as conference leader makes the arrangements for the conference and establishes the objectives. The leader may be the primary nurse, if this is the system used in the hospital, or it may be the head nurse or supervisor. The leader must be someone who is familiar with the patient's problem. Only those persons directly involved in care of the patient should be included in the meeting. The appropriate time and place must be established, just as in any meeting.

Patient care conferences are often conducted in the room designated for shift reports and charting. The number of persons included should be limited to allow for more open discussion. One person should record the discussion during the conference and document the facts on the patient's chart. When patient care conferences are held routinely at specified times on the nursing unit, fewer arrangements are necessary. There may be follow-up conferences with progress reports if the patient is hospitalized for a relatively long period of time.

Example of a Patient Care Conference

As an example of a called patient care conference, Mr. Bender was the primary nurse for Mr. Sutton, an 82-year-old man with pneumonia. He was responding well to treatment but refused to get out of bed. His wife stayed with him during the day and did everything for him. She had expressed her fear of his becoming worse from doing too much. Mr. Bender had tried various methods to get Mr. Sutton up and had explained the importance of mobility to Mrs. Sutton, but nothing had been effective. He decided to call a patient care conference with the head nurse, the evening nurse, the physical therapist, and the wife in attendance. The meeting was scheduled for 1330 for minimum interference with work routines.

Mr. Bender opened the conference by stating the objectives of Mr. Sutton remaining out of bed for progressively longer periods of time and gradually increasing ambulation. The head nurse explained to Mrs. Sutton the importance of mobility and ambulation. Various ideas were discussed, including a positive approach toward Mr. Sutton. The physical therapist was requested to assist Mr. Sutton in his initial ambulation. After realizing the importance of getting her husband out of bed, Mrs. Sutton suggested removing the urinal from the bedside during the day and insisting that Mr. Sutton go to the bathroom. It was also agreed that all meals would be taken while sitting in a chair. A follow-up conference was scheduled for 5 days later with the head nurse, primary nurse, and Mrs. Sutton.

All concerned were pleased with the results. Mr. Sutton was staying out of bed 3 to 4 hours a day, walking to the nurses' desk and back twice a day, and looking forward to discharge. The patient care conference had enabled all persons responsible for Mr. Sutton's care to work together to maximize care.

Routine Conferences

Sometimes patient care conferences are on a routine basis. The patient presented at the conference may be one requested by a nurse, or nurses may be assigned to present a patient on a designated date. As an example, on an oncology unit one nurse is responsible for conducting a conference each week. During this meeting the patient's response to treatment and the stages of grief exhibited by the patient and family are discussed. All of the staff nurses contribute to the discussion and share similar experiences, noting approaches that were found to be effective with other patients. This enables the nurse presenting the meeting to more effectively assist the patient and the family in coping with the situation and often gives the nurse the support needed to deal with oncology nursing.

Shift Reports

Reports at each change of shift are vital to continuity of care of patients. There are several methods of presenting shift reports.

Oral and Taped Reports

One method is for the charge nurse on the outgoing shift to report on all of the patients to the entire oncoming shift. This is probably more effective on small nursing units where the staff is familiar with all or most of the patients. Occasionally the report is given by the charge nurse of the preceding shift to the oncoming charge nurse, who then relays the information to each primary nurse or team. This prevents nurses who are involved in direct care from validating information and is not generally recommended.

The report may include all patients and may be taped by the charge nurse with the oncoming staff listening as a group. Each primary nurse may give an oral or a taped report on the assigned patients to all of the oncoming shift or only to those who will be responsible for the same patients. Taped reports have a disadvantage in that the nurses who are listening are not able to ask questions during the report. Sometimes they may make inquiries following the report, but the information desired may have been forgotten and is not as meaningful as when the report is being given.

Clinical Rounds

Another method of giving a shift report is the "walking report" or clinical rounds, in which nurses from each shift make patient rounds together. The charge nurse may give the report only to the charge nurse of the oncoming shift, or the primary nurses may give a report to the charge nurse and to those who will be responsible for the same patients on the next shift. These rounds may be given at the bedside with the patient as a participant. In this instance the nurse must be prepared to answer any questions the patient may have.

More frequently the information is given outside of the patient's room, with a brief visit to the bedside by both nurses. This method is very effective because the oncoming nurse is able to briefly visit with each patient and ask any questions of the nurse on the previous shift. There may be various combinations used in shift reports. The two charge nurses may make clinical rounds, with oncoming primary nurses or teams receiving verbal or taped reports from the outgoing shift.

Setting

Regardless of the method of shift report, there are details that make any report more effective. One factor is the place where the report is given. It must be private, away from patients, and where there will be no distractions outside of emergencies. Most nursing units have a nurses' lounge or break room that is used for reports. It may be necessary to give a shift report at the nurses' station, but this should be avoided if at all possible.

During report, nurses on the outgoing shift should be assigned to answer phones, lights, and take care of any requests that might arise. A factor to keep in mind when giving a report on a series of patients is that a logical order should be followed. Numerical sequence of rooms is the order most frequently used.

Information to Include

A good shift report gives a concise, complete picture of the patient's condition. It contains all pertinent facts and omits extraneous details that do not contribute to patient care. All of the information should be exact—the specific medication or treatment, the time of occurrence, and the precise behavior of the patient, for example.

Any report should start with the patient's name and exact room and bed location. It is helpful to follow this with the patient's age, doctor, admission diagnosis, and any surgery performed. This refreshes the memory of those who were working the previous day and gives the needed information to those who were not. Tests that have been done in the past 24 hours and results, if known, should be included. The general condition of the patient and any changes in health status since the previous day, whether an improvement or deterioration, should be noted. Changes in orders such as medication changes or laboratory tests or X-rays to be performed must be relayed to the next shift to minimize errors.

Nursing diagnoses are an integral part of a shift report. Reviewing the nursing diagnoses and adding any new ones stresses the nursing concerns. Reports should include nursing orders for meeting the needs of the patient as reflected in the diagnoses. Nursing interventions should be evaluated with recommendations to continue or to change. Emotional status is often a factor in determining nursing interventions; any unmet emotional needs should be incorporated into the nursing diagnoses to enable the nurse on the next shift to more effectively care for the patient.

Items That Should Be Included in a Shift Report on a Patient

Patient's name, age, sex, room, and bed
Doctor and admission diagnosis
Surgery and/or diagnostic tests

General status and any change
Any new or changed physicians' orders
Nursing diagnoses and suggested interventions or nursing orders
Evaluation of nursing interventions

Example of a Shift Report

A typical shift report at the end of the day shift on one patient might be as follows.

> Mrs. Burnham, in Room 422, Bed B, is a 66-year-old women who was admitted by Dr. Sanders today with a medical diagnosis of cholelithiasis. She complained of RUQ pain on admission, which was relieved by 50 mg of Demerol at 1145. A cholecystogram is scheduled for tomorrow. The prep medication has been ordered but not received from the pharmacy. Medication orders are for Demerol 50 mg prn and Dalmane at HS. One nursing order is to monitor for comfort as specified by the nursing diagnosis of alteration in comfort: RUQ pain related to cholelithiasis. The nursing diagnosis of fear related to possibility of surgery suggests finding time for interpersonal communication this evening.

From this information the nurses on the oncoming shift have a clear, concise picture of the patient's admission problem and current status to facilitate planning the evening care routine. Any further questions they might have can be clarified if the report is presented orally. This same format should be followed when giving a report on several patients.

Communication among members of the health care team is essential to quality patient care. In an open exchange of information, problem areas can be discovered that would not be apparent to some members of the team. Measures can then be instituted so that health care personnel can work together toward a solution. Communication among health care personnel helps each team member to see patients as individuals with unique backgrounds and current needs. This promotes personalizing care and establishes better communication by every team member with the patient.

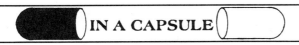

IN A CAPSULE

Effective *nurse to nurse communication* is enhanced by self-acceptance, expression of emotions, and a degree of assertiveness. It is important to remain in control of emotions in any *superior/subordinate communication*, regardless of the position. The nurse is responsible for establishing an atmosphere of mutual respect in *communication with aides*. *Student/ staff communication* usually places the staff nurse in the superior position, but one in which productive experiences are promoted for the student.

Problems seen in *nurse-physician communication* stemming from the *evolving role of the nurse can be solved through reciprocally open communication. Interdisciplinary team communication* has gained attention as the various health care givers are becoming more involved in planning and evaluating patient care.

Written records are invaluable for communication with the health care team, as educational tools, for research and statistics, to monitor quality of care, and as legal documentation. The form of *patient charts* varies but includes the physicians' orders, history, physical, and progress notes, the reports and record of treatments of all ancillary departments, and the nurses' medication records, assessments, and notes of care given. Some *written memos* are not a part of the patient charts but include requisitions to various departments and reminders or points of concern to physicians and other health care personnel.

Patient records are considered *legal documents* and are used to verify charges, to audit quality of care, as a narcotic check, and as prime evidence in any litigation. Personal information received from patients during the course of care is considered *privileged communication* and should be shared only if directly related to health status.

Planned *nursing team communication* is accomplished through patient care plans, patient care conferences, and shift reports. *Patient care conferences* should involve those directly involved in the care of the patient and/or the current problem. A good *shift report* gives a clear, concise report of all pertinent facts contributing to the patient's current status with no extraneous data.

DO YOU REMEMBER

- factors that promote effective communication between nurses?
- a responsibility of the nurse in communicating with aides?
- the communication level of the nurse with other health care professionals?
- advantages of interdisciplinary team communication?
- the purpose of written patient records?
- general information included in patient charts?
- where incident and accident reports are filed and why?
- some actions by the nurse that decrease the chance of a malpractice suit?
- planned methods of nursing team communication?

CAN YOU DESCRIBE

- the manner in which potentially uncomfortable superior/subordinate interactions can be avoided?
- relationships that you as a student nurse have had with a staff nurse?
- factors contributing to and ramifications of the "doctor/nurse game"?
- written memos related to patient care that are not a part of the patient chart?
- elements that comprise an effective shift report?

ACTION, PLEASE

1. Work with another student to give a shift report on a patient who has recently been assigned to you. Use any notes you have available. Have the other student check to determine the inclusion of pertinent information without any unnecessary data. Reverse roles.

2. Consider the following patient information.

Mrs. Davis was hospitalized with a fever of unknown origin. While he was being cared for, he frequently talked of his personal life. He was married and had three teen-age children. He stated that he had been taking antacids regularly because his wife's constant nagging was giving him ulcers. He had recently spent several weekends, including the preceding one, with another woman in a mountain resort in Colorado. He did not want to divorce his wife because of the children but was afraid the other woman was pregnant. Mr. Davis mentioned having removed several ticks from the two of them while in Colorado. You are aware that several febrile conditions can be caused by tick bites.

Hopefully, you will not be confronted with a situation of this magnitude, but it is always possible. In light of the fact that Mr. Davis has had an elevated temperature, note the manner in which you would handle the information received.

a. Exactly what would you chart?

_____

_____

_____

b. What would you share verbally with other health care personnel?

_____

_____

_____

c. With which specific health professionals would you share the preceding information?

_____

_____

_____

d. What would you not share with anyone?

_____

_____

_____

3. *How Would You Organize This Patient Care Conference?* Mrs. Matthews has been hospitalized for 4 weeks following a stroke. Her husband and daughters have been taking turns staying with her. She has not responded to therapy as rapidly as the doctor thinks she should and will not attempt to do anything for herself.

a. Who would you include in the conference?

_____

_____

b. How would you arrange the time and place?

_____

_____

c. What would be the objectives?

_____

_____

d. How would you conduct the conference?

_____

_____

e. What would you record and where?

_____

_____

f. Would you arrange a follow-up conference? If so, when?

_____

_____

_____

11

Nurses'
Documentation of
Patient Care

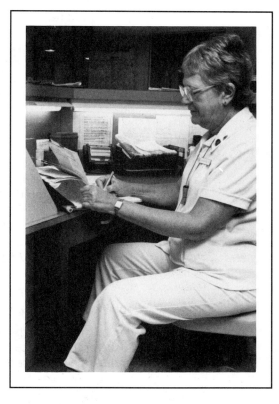

The thinking you do before you start a job will shorten the time you take to spend working on it.
Roy L. Smith

OBJECTIVES

Upon completion of this chapter, the student will be able to:

- discuss the significance of using correct medical terminology.
- give reasons for the limited use of medical terms with patients.
- note precautions in the use of abbreviations.
- describe the categories of information that nurses record.
- discuss application of principles of charting in documenting patient care.
- list items required or restricted for nurses' notes to be technically correct.
- state application and limitation of narrative-style documentation.
- explain the emphasis and advantages in problem-oriented charting.
- differentiate the formats used in prob-

229

lem-oriented records.
- construct nurses' progress notes from a given situation using the narrative style and one or more of the problem-oriented formats.
- discuss advantages and disadvantages in the use of flow sheets.
- list ways in which the nurse can reduce charting time.
- explore possibilities in the use of computers in documenting patient care.

GLOSSARY OF TERMS*

Narrative style   In no particular order, as in telling a story.

Objective   Facts without distortion by personal feelings or bias; derived from sense perception or scientific measurement; verifiable by others.

Problem oriented   Arranged in preset order and directed toward a particular problem.

Subjective   Pertaining to reality as perceived; not perceived by senses or verifiable.

Telegraphic style   Written with economy of words; concise; terse.

*Definitions applicable to content.

Written communication with the health care team in general has been discussed. The focus of this chapter is the nurses' written documentation of patient care. Nurses' notes include facets of daily care, observations by the nurse, and evaluation of the response of the patient to medical and nursing interventions. The nurses' written record is essential from the standpoint of continuity of care as well as the legal consideration of proof of care given.

IMPORTANCE OF CORRECT MEDICAL TERMINOLOGY

Most fields of endeavor develop a language specific to the discipline. In any field it is essential to use correct terms with co-workers for better understanding. A general knowledge of medical terminology enables various departments within a health care facility to communicate more effectively.

Without a medical vocabulary, communication among nurses would be difficult. What would the primary nurse think if a student described a patient as "looking a funny color, breathing weird, and sort of jerking around"? The ability of the student would no doubt be questioned. To describe a papular rash on the abdomen as "funny red bumps on the stomach" might get a laugh but certainly would not be considered a proper assessment. The use of correct terminology reduces the amount of time required to send a message and gives an accurate picture to the other health care worker.

Developing a Medical Vocabulary

It is essential that students develop an adequate vocabulary for charting. An awareness of components of medical terms helps to determine meanings of vaguely familiar words. New terms are presented in conjunction with each new concept in the nursing program. These should become a part of the student's vocabulary when studied.

Developing the habit of consulting a dictionary when any unfamiliar terms are encountered will strengthen the student's active medical vocabulary. If unsure of which term to use when charting, the student should look it up in a text or ask an instructor or experienced nurse. The meaning of a term should never be guessed. Terms should not be used just because they appear in earlier notes on the chart.

Use of Clinical Terms with Patients

It is important to use correct medical terminology with the health care team, but medical "jargon" may leave patients confused at a time when they most need to know what is happening. A few patients may know enough medical terminology to understand the words, but most will not. The patient finds no reassurance in a garble of technical terms. This only leads to more feelings of fear and insecurity and elevates an already high level of anxiety.

Why do nurses use technical terms with patients? It may be a verbal smoke screen that avoids the challenge of plain language. It may be from insensitivity to the patient's or family's needs. It may make the speaker feel more detached from the situation by using impersonal technical terms. Patients often hesitate to ask for medical terms to be explained in understandable terms for fear of being labeled ignorant.

The general public is exposed to more health education and the use of technical terms through television and the press than in the past, but the average person's medical vocabulary is still limited. Use of clinical terms can result in unnecessary anxiety as well as lack of compliance when directions are not understood. Nurses should assess the patient's level of understanding of medical terms and use only those they are certain the patient understands.

Effective communication is essential for patient satisfaction in health care received, and understandable language is essential to effective communication. The nurse who has a strong basic medical vocabulary is able to convert medical terms to language easily understood by the patient more readily than a person who has only vague ideas of the meaning of the terms.

Abbreviations: Usage and Dangers

Abbreviations are timesaving devices used for everything from reports in a large corporation to special abbreviations for a grocery list. In health care agencies, abbreviations are used rather extensively. Some of these are generally accepted, some are seen in specific areas of the country, some are within a particular institution, and some are only used in certain specialty units. Each health care facility has a list of abbreviations that are acceptable in it.

Medical abbreviations can be misinterpreted or misread. For example, in one instance the doctor had ordered "H & H q AM." This was interpreted as half and half, so the patient was given a glass of half milk and half cream. When the doctor made rounds, he was very perturbed because the lab had not completed a hemoglobin and hematocrit. This kind of mistake can lead to serious errors.

Some of the errors related to abbreviations may be attributed to handwriting. In an atmosphere in which personnel are constantly pressed for time, medical personnel may not take the time to write legibly. This compounds the interpretation of abbreviations as well as written drug names. Names of medications should never be abbreviated. Many orders for times and routes of administration of medications use abbreviations that are generally accepted but may be illegible. The use of both metric and apothecary measures further complicates interpretation. Whenever there is any doubt about a physician's order, the nurse should question it.

The use of computers to enter new or changed orders has been suggested as a solution to the misinterpretation of physicians' handwritten orders. This might be more time-consuming for the doctor when first instituted but would eliminate many errors. Physicians, however, are often resistant to the idea.

Abbreviations are used frequently in nurses' notes. Many are acceptable, but the use can be carried to extremes in documentation. What does "Dr. May vs. LOC ordered" mean? These abbreviations may be accepted in some institutions to mean, "Dr. May visited. Laxative of choice ordered." In other health care facilities the abbreviation form would not be acceptable since LOC is more often considered to mean level of consciousness. The nurse should always check the list accepted in the facility before charting and use only those abbreviations included on the list. When in doubt, the entry should be written out.

CHECK IT OUT

Find the list of accepted abbreviations on your clinical unit. This may take a bit of searching, but it should be available. Look through some charts for unfamiliar abbreviations.

Check to see it they are on the accepted list.

GENERAL FACTORS IN DOCUMENTATION OF PATIENT CARE

The nurses' progress record, or nurses' notes, is an important aspect of patient care. Many nurses complain about the amount of paper work involved, stating that it takes valuable time that they feel would be better spent at the bedside. This may seem a logical complaint, but how would continuity or quality care be maintained without documentation?

Another aspect to consider is the legal implications. How would a nurse prove that adequate care had been delivered without a record? Well-written notes do take time and require knowledge and skill in writing, but a good chart defends itself in the clinical setting and in a legal situation. Professional charting reflects professional care. Correct terminology must be used if charting is to be accepted as professional.

The following principles of charting must be combined with the accountability of the nurse to present the current status of the client. Awareness of the importance of documentation should prevent it from becoming a chore and an exercise in futility.

Categories of Information Recorded by Nurses

In general, information that the nurse documents can be classified as observations and actions. The observations can be grouped into objective and subjective data.

Objective Data

Objective data recorded by the nurse includes anything that is observed through the senses—that which is seen, heard, felt, or smelled. It is also any data, such as vital signs, that can be measured by means of an instrument. All objective data can be verified by other persons. Objective data does not involve drawing conclusions or analyzing data. It is simply facts.

Objective data recorded by the nurse specifically describes overt patient behaviors, the physical status of the patient with technically correct descriptions, and any measurements taken, ranging from vital signs to size of decubitus. There is no place for the nurse's conclusions in charting. Although the nurse may think that the patient is depressed, only the observed, overt behavior is charted.

Subjective Data

Subjective data is information the nurse receives in ways other than those mentioned in the preceding paragraphs. Anything the patient or family tells the nurse is subjective data. It cannot be measured with an instrument or determined through any of the nurses' senses. It could include pain, fear, anxiety, and all other emotional aspects of responses. There may be physical, observable indications of the presence of pain, but the pain itself is not visible.

When the information recorded is subjective, it should be indicated as such on the chart by using quotation marks or noting, "states . . ." The subjective data includes any complaints of the patient, misunderstandings the patient might verbalize, or pertinent questions by the patient, such as requesting information about a procedure.

Actions of the Nurse

The other category of data recorded by the nurse is actions. This includes the implementation of daily hygienic measures, various therapies, and any related activities. Patient response to nursing actions is part of the recording. Responses and/or evaluations recorded are objective and subjective data. The nurse records actual care given as well as any information imparted in patient teaching. Notification of a superior regarding the status of the patient or an unusual incident should be included. When reporting any information to the physician's office, the person who received the information should be noted. The nurse may record observed actions of other members of the health team, such as, "Dressing changed by Dr. Smith."

CHECK IT OUT

Read the following entries made on a chart. Determine which are subjective, objective, or conclusions drawn by the nurse.

> States did not sleep well.
> Eyes red from crying.
> Turned to left side.
> Very anxious regarding surgery.
> My back is really hurting.

Small abrasion left forearm.
Ambulated in hall unassisted.
Check with classmates. Do you agree?

Principles of Recording Nurses' Progress Notes

Nurses' progress notes reflect what is done for patients, how they are protected, and how their property is protected. Nursing notes reflect patients' daily progress and emotional, as well as physical, adjustment to their current status. Nurses' notes should reflect the plan of care that has been designed for that particular individual. There are basic rules that apply to making entries on the patient chart. These may vary somewhat from one agency to another but are essentially the same. Entries should be accurate, complete, factual, clear, appropriate, concise, current, and technically correct.

Accurate

Any notations made by the nurse must be accurate and specific in time, amounts, descriptions, and responses. The 24-hour clock, or military time, is used in many institutions to avoid the possibility of confusing AM and PM. Thus 1200 is noon and 2400 midnight; 0900 is 9:00 AM and 2100 is 9:00 PM. Medical terms and accepted abbreviations should be used in describing any signs and symptoms or behaviors. For accurate descriptions, specific terms should be used. What does "Had a good night" mean? Good compared to what? When a note states, "Condition improved today," what is meant? Is the patient ready for discharge? Or has the patient just been taken off the critical list? When charting dietary intake, does "ate well" mean anything? State the approximate percentage of food eaten, such as, "Ate 50% regular diet." Relative statements do not tell to what they are related. Observations that are charted should give an accurate picture of the situation.

All entries on charts should be made *after* the procedure has been completed, unless recording a plan for action. The nurse may plan to carry out a procedure or give a medication, but any number of things can interrupt the plan. If nurses sometimes chart before completing a nursing action and this fact is known, the credibility of the nurses' notes will be questioned. Deliberately making inaccurate entries on a chart can lead to civil or criminal charges with the possibility of losing the license to practice nursing. This holds true of any data that is purposely omitted, because an omission is considered an inaccuracy. All entries must be truthful and include the facts as known by the nurse.

Correct spelling is essential if a record is to be considered accurate. Incorrect spelling of technical terms can completely change the meaning. To state that a patient is dysphasic when the difficulty is in swallowing makes the entire statement inaccurate, even though only one letter is wrong. Dysphasia means difficulty in speech, while dysphagia indicates difficulty in swallowing. One notation on a chart referred to the "public area" instead of the "pubic area."

Incorrect spelling of nontechnical terms is sometimes seen on charts. To read that a patient is unable to "here" well or that a medication is refused because of "fear of addition" makes nurses' notes a source of amusement. Misspelled words can cause misunderstandings as well as convey an unprofessional image to others. If nurses' notes were projected on the wall of a courtroom (as they often are in a trial) with misspelled words, the professionalism and credibility of the nurse would be questioned. If these examples seem far fetched, random samples of entries on charts should be read.

Complete

It is essential to record *all* pertinent data with no omissions of information on the condition of the patient, even though some notes may simply state that the findings are normal. Recording this fact indicates that the observations have been made. Certain items are universally required in nursing documentation. An admission assessment and a discharge summary are usually on form sheets. When a patient returns to the unit from a diagnostic procedure or surgery, the time and condition are recorded.

Accidents or unusual incidents have been discussed. If a patient refuses a medication or treatment, this should be noted with the reason for refusal. "I am not going to take that medicine. It makes me feel too lightheaded," accurately tells why the medication was refused. The status of the patient, any changes in physical functioning, signs and symptoms that are severe or recurring, and any behavioral changes are worthy of notation. Visits of family and friends are often recorded. Some agencies prefer that the nurse note the visits of the doctor and other health professionals and any of their procedures observed.

What a nurse does not chart can be detrimental. An incomplete chart suggests incomplete nursing care. Many health care facilities require a complete assessment of the patient at least once a day, others on each shift. Long-term care facilities and agencies providing home health care vary in these requirements, some using a daily or a shift focus to record different aspects of the patients' status each day.

Nurses protect themselves by recording assessments at the beginning and end of the shift. This assessment specifically states the condition of the patient when care began and ended. This may be time-consuming at first, but with use of this approach, techniques are developed that enable the nurse to complete the assessment and recording in minimal time.

Complete charting can make a difference in Medicare payments. If the signs, symptoms, and response to treatment are adequately recorded, Medicare often will make payments even though the diagnosis indicated by the symptoms has not been specifically stated on the chart.

Factual

Information recorded by the nurse must be factual. Factual information can be verified by others. It is objective observations, and these observations should be stated specifically. The conclusions of the nurse are not objective statements and should never be a part of the chart. The words "appears to be . . ," "apparently . . ," or "seems . . ." should not appear in the nurses' notes. These notations indicate interpretations or conclusions drawn by the nurse. The only time "appears to be . . ." can ever be considered acceptable is when the patient is apparently sleeping. This, too, can be avoided by stating that the patient is lying quietly with eyes closed.

The nurse may believe that the patient is depressed, but the chart should reflect only the behaviors observed. The notes may read, "Refuses to talk except to give short answers. Sitting in chair in slumped position." Others may draw the same conclusion from the behaviors noted, but it is possible that the patient is tired or experiencing some discomfort. Behaviors should be accurately described without labeling the patient or the cause of the particular behaviors.

Subjective data described by the patient should be charted, but the fact that they are subjective should be qualified. The patient will disclose many symptoms. Those that are not observable must be recorded to indicate that they were the patient's description. "States severe pain left knee," is a factual statement since it notes that the patient said it. If the patient complains of an itching back, inspection might reveal a rash. This could be charted, "C/O back itching. Numerous wheals noted over upper back. Dr. Turner notified." This notes the patient's complaint, the nurse's actions in response to it, and the fact that the complaint was called to the doctor's attention. The only subjective data is the complaint of the patient, which is identified as such. The remainder is objective data.

Clear

Any language used in charting should be readily understandable to others. Ambiguous terms should not be used, and the abbreviations accepted by the institution should be adhered to. Run-on sentences or wording that is difficult to understand should be avoided. Following are some examples of charting that could easily be misinterpreted.

> Prostate exam by Dr. Fine on floor.
> Complained about left elbow on admission but it has disappeared today.
> When pain is relieved, it is not entirely relieved.
> When you pin him down, he has some lower abdomen pain.

These notes might bring a chuckle, but cannot be recommended. The nurse should be aware of the manner in which notes are worded so that they will not be misunderstood. The correct terminology to adequately describe the patient's status should be used. Instead of "unable to bend left elbow very far," "limited flexion left elbow" should be charted. Instead of "sweating a large amount," "profuse diaphoresis" should be the entry. Instead of "watery drainage with some blood," "serosanguineous drainage" would be the better choice. Use of correct terminology is essential to professional charting.

Appropriate

Information recorded in the nurses' notes must be appropriate and deal with the current status of the patient. As noted, the nurse receives information from the patient that is not relevant to health status. This data has no place in the chart. Other "garbage," or unnecessary information, should not be given space in the chart. It is unnecessary to chart "linen changed," since this is considered a part of routine morning care. The only time it would be appropriate is when changing linen is not a part of routine care, as with an incontinent patient. If flow sheets are used, the information should not be repeated in the nurses' progress notes. However, if there is an abnormal assessment noted on the flow sheet, this should be documented fully.

Concise

Nurses' notes should be brief and to the point. Only what is important should be recorded. Health personnel reading the chart for an update on the status of the patient are not intersted in flowery descriptions and a lengthy discourse but want to get the facts in the shortest possible length of time. Contrary to what is taught during the school years, complete sentences are not recommended in nurses' notes. Most institutions prefer what is termed "telegraphic" style. When sending a telegram, there is a charge for every word. Therefore, the message is conveyed in as few words as possible. This is the manner in which nurses' notes should be written to reduce space and reading time. It consists of short phrases rather than complete sentences. It is usually best to begin each phrase with a capital letter and end it with a period. Compare the following entries.

> Patient C/O having a headache and requested pain medical for relief.
> C/O headache. Requested pain medication.

The meaning is the same, but the second one requires less writing and reading time.

Most agencies do not require or want the name of the patient in entries or the word "patient" or "client" in notations. It is assumed that anything recorded on Mr. Brown's chart refers to him and not to Mr. Green. There will be instances when it is acceptable for the sake of clarity to include the word "patient." When talking with patient and family together or with family members regarding the patient, there must be a means to convey which information was contributed by each. For example:

> Patient and wife instructed on dressing change. Patient expressed doubt regarding ability to perform procedure. Wife demonstrated dressing change without difficulty.

This documents patient teaching and denotes responses of the two persons involved. Chart entries should be made in as few words as possible to accurately describe the situation.

Current

Nurses' notes must be kept current. There are some items that can wait for a break to be charted, such as relatively routine care and daily assessments when there are no acute problems. However, any medications, complaints of pain, or unusual events should be recorded immediately. The chart must be current before the nurse leaves the unit for any reason. For example, consider the following situation. Miss Brown has just given a patient a medication for pain and needs to pick up some solution for a wet dressing. The pharmacy is on the same floor, so she decides to pick up the solution before charting. There are several nurses waiting for the pharmacist, and her short absence lengthens. She returns to the unit to find another nurse preparing a second dose of the pain medication. Charting the pain medication immediately would have averted this "near error."

Health care agencies differ in policies regarding how often entries must be made in the nurses' notes. Some require notations every hour, some every 2 hours, and some each shift. Some long-term care facilities chart only daily. The stated policy should be followed. However, care should be taken to include all necessary information. To ensure timeliness in recording items that do not need to be charted immediately, a notebook may be carried in the pocket for personal notes. This not only ensures noting the correct times but also guards against any omission in notations.

Technically Correct

This phrase covers a number of aspects of charting. A page of nurses' notes is not accepted as legal evidence if it is not technically correct. This requires meeting the following criteria.

1. Each page must have the patient's name and identification number on it.

2. Each entry must have the date and time noted.

3. The person documenting the care must sign the entry with first initial, last name, and abbreviation indicating status, for example, RN, LPN, etc. Some agencies require the full name rather than the first initial. There may be one signature for several entries if there are no intervening entries.

4. Nurses should chart only the care that they have given. Nurses cannot chart for other nurses or ask others to chart for them. If it is necessary to make notations for another nurse, this should be indicated in the notes. For example, Martha Johnson called in to say that she had forgotten to make a notation on a patient during her shift. The notation should state, "0730 M. Johnson called. Reported administered Fleet's enema at 0600 . . ." Martha should check the notation the next night and sign it if correct or make a correction if not.

5. If the agency requires a countersignature, the nurse should check the care given and review the entry before countersigning. Some institutions require that an RN countersign all entries by student nurses or aides. The nurse countersigning an entry is accepting responsibility for the accurate assessment or completion of the procedure charted.

6. There should be no blank lines or spaces. This is a safeguard for the person entering the data, since someone could enter false information in any space left blank, or the blank space could be interpreted as intention to fill it in at a later time.

7. All entries should be in chronological order. If a nurse has failed to make an entry on time, it may be entered later by noting the date and time with "late entry" before the data charted. The entry should be cross-referenced with the page on which it was omitted if on a different page.

8. Erasures, whiteouts, or blackouts are not legally acceptable. If an error is made, a single line should be drawn through the entry and "error" noted with initials. The incorrect entry must be legible after correction. It is easy to pick up the wrong chart and start to make an entry before the mistake is realized. The nurse should make a habit of checking the name on the chart before starting to make an entry, since charts can be placed in the wrong slot in the rack. If copying a page of nurses' notes, it should be stated that it is a copy. The original should be filed with the chart.

9. Ditto marks are never acceptable on a chart, even though the entry reads the same as the entry above.

10. Nurses' notes must be legible. Printing or cursive writing is acceptable but must be legible to be technically correct.

11. All documentation on the patient chart must be in ink. Institutions vary in the color of ink that is used. Some use different colors on each shift, and some require all entries to be in black.

This discussion of the principles of documenting patient care may make the process seem complicated. The telegraphic style may be different from that to which a nurse is accustomed, but the nurse may find it easier than writing in grammatically correct complete sentences. Many instructors require that students submit a rough draft of notes to be reviewed before writing them on the chart. Even experienced nurses often make a rough draft if the situation they are documenting is somewhat unusual.

It is always acceptable to ask another's opinion if in doubt about wording on a chart. Charting becomes easier with practice, so the student should not be discouraged if it seems difficult at first. Only when the nurses' notes reflect care given and the patient's current status will documentation serve to provide the intended purposes.

CHECK IT OUT

Look at the following brief nurses' notes. Determine whether they follow the principles in the preceding paragraphs. If not, what is wrong with each one? Restate to make correct.

1. Patient slept well all night.
2. Seems depressed.
3. Mrs. Evans said that she would like to have some medication for the pain in her left arm.
4. Frowning. Hands tightly clenched.
5. Dr. Green saw patient while on floor.

FORMAT OF NURSES' DOCUMENTATION OF CARE

The manner in which nurses' progress notes are written and the forms on which the entries are made will vary in different health care facilities. The same principles basically apply, regardless of the format used. If these principles are learned as a student and conscientiously applied, there should be no problem in adapting to the guidelines in any institution. The more commonly used formats will be considered, although there may be variations of these in different agencies. No one way is considered "right," so all entries should be made according to the policy of the institution.

Narrative Style

Narrative charting is sometimes termed traditional, since it is an older style that has been in use for years in nursing. Many health care agencies still use this format.

It does not follow a particular order except that the notes are chronologically recorded, but the same information will be seen on narrative notes as on any other style.

These notes contain patient assessments, nursing interventions and patient responses, specific measures carried out by the physician, visits by members of the health care team, and any other significant information. Items such as specimens or requisitions sent to the laboratory and the time the patient leaves or returns to the unit are often noted. The notes are written in telegraphic style, adhering to the principles discussed. If properly written, this type of format can be effective. However, it does not usually indicate the nursing diagnoses and care plan.

Figure 11.1 is an example of narrative notes for Mrs. Stevens, who had abdominal surgery 3 days ago and is recuperating without any special problems. She complained of pain in area of incision at 0930 and received medication that relieved the pain.

0800	Awake, alert, oriented x 3. PERLA. Eupneic. Lung sounds clear. Pulse strong, regular all extremities. Skin pink, warm, dry. No edema noted. Abd. dressing dry & intact. No other skin lesions noted. Ambulates to bath by self. Denies pain or discomfort. ——————————
0930	C/O dull pain in incisional area. Frowning, holding abd. Requested oral pain med. Tylenol #3 P.O. ——————————————————————————— J. Duffy, RN
1015	States pain relieved. ————————————————————————— J. Duffy, RN

Figure 11.1: Narrative nurses' notes.

The date would be noted at the top of the page if a separate page is used each day or at the point at which the first entry after midnight was made. The 0800 assessment was essentially normal, the kind that can wait for a break to record. Therefore, this entry is not signed, since it was made at the same time as the 0930 entry. Much of the assessment data would be omitted if on a flow sheet, and some additional information might be included in this entry if routine care was not included on a flow sheet. The 0930 entry reflects the status of the patient and the nursing intervention with the evaluation of the action noted at 1015. Note that telegraphic style is used for the notes. This same information can be recorded using another format, as will be seen in the next section.

Problem-Oriented Records

The problem-oriented medical record (POMR) was introduced in the 1960's by Dr. Weed as a patient-centered approach to charting. It was originally developed for all health care personnel to chart on a continuous progress record. Thus, reading straight through a chart would give a chronological record of the patient's treatment and progress. The problem-oriented medical record is currently used in many health care agencies in this or, more often, a modified form. Separate pages frequently are used for progress notes for the various health care personnel such as physicians, nurses, various therapists, dietitians, etc. This approach is aimed toward problem solving. The general format of the nurses' progress record is the same, regardless of whether the departments are integrated in progress record entries or separated.

Data Base

There is always a data base in problem-oriented records that contains the information received from the patient or family on admission. The data base also includes information from the nursing assessment and history, medical assessment and physical examination notes of the physician, laboratory and X-ray data, and any additional social and family information from other sources.

Problem List

A problem list denotes any areas of concern assessed from analysis of the data. The manner in which the problem list is created varies. The initial problem list may be made by the physician, with the nurses and other members of the health care team adding areas of concern noted. Some facilities use a problem list with sublists. The main problem reflects a medical diagnosis, while the sublists are nursing diagnoses related to the medical diagnosis. In other agencies, there are separate lists of medical and nursing problems. Physicians in some hospitals do not follow the problem-oriented approach, but the nurses' documentation is a problem-oriented format.

Some agencies place only active problems on the list. Potential problems may be part of the problem list, or they may be noted on the progress record and placed on the problem list only when they become active. Sometimes inactive problems remain on the list for alerting the staff to the possibility of recurrence or as a type of summary. The problems in the list are usually numbered for reference in progress notes.

Plans

Plans are then made to work toward solution of the problems. These are overall plans. The physician's plans note what is to be done first, indicating the priority of the identified problems. Sometimes the physician writes orders numbered according to the problem each addresses. The plans include not only the therapy ordered by the physician but also plans written by the nurse, such as nursing care plans or plans of other health team members. Patient education should be included in the list of plans.

Progress Records

Progress records are an integral part of the problem-oriented health record. Notes are made by all members of the health care team involved in care of the patient. The notations may all be on the same record or on separate ones. The SOAP format is used for recording progress. This is the reason problem-oriented charting is frequently referred to as "soaping notes."

> **S Subjective data** includes what patients state, what they perceive, and the way they express it. Emotional responses are included in this data only if specifically expressed by the patient, such as, "I am really mad about the way I was treated."

O Objective data includes observations made through the use any of the senses or measurements by instruments of any kind. This data can be verified by other people.

A Assessments are made based on the preceding data. Team members make these assessments based on their special knowledge and field of experience. Conclusions are drawn regarding the interpretation of the data. This requires a knowledge base as well as logical thinking. Nursing diagnoses are often entered here.

P Plans are made to resolve the problem noted in the assessment. The plan may be of a therapeutic, educational, or diagnostic nature. Plans are based on the data, which may indicate a problem that needs attention, a lack of knowledge or skills necessary for self-care, or a need to explore further to obtain additional data.

If the SOAP charting stops at this step, the notes do not actually state that the plan has been implemented, even though it is assumed. Some institutions use a SOAPIE format, adding two steps to the SOAP format above.

I The **implementation** records what is actually done, not just planned. These entries are specific as to details of what the nurse actually did.

E Evaluation of the patient's response may be included in the notes. This indicates whether or not the action was effective. The evaluation should be stated in terms of the patient's behavior or words.

There may be an "R" added to the preceding. It is then referred to as a SOAPIER format.

R Revision may be necessary if the plan used was not effective. There may be changes in the patient's condition that warrant a review of previous plans.

Health care agencies will vary in the manner in which the problem-oriented charting system is applied. Some form of the SOAPIER format of recording patient progress is usually used. The problem number is often referred to with each entry. Many agencies do not require that each step be included in all entries. There may be only subjective and objective items recorded if the data does not indicate the need for a nursing intervention. Each institution will have reasons for the particular application. No one way is right or wrong.

In the section on narrative notations, we looked at Mrs. Stevens, who was 3 days post-op following abdominal surgery with no acute problems. In Figure 11.2 the same information is recorded in a SOAPIE format.

The information is the same as in the narrative format but entered little differently. The information in "O" will vary according to flow charts used, and the "E" may be timed separately. Both methods adhere to the principles of charting discussed, except that in the SOAP format a plan is included rather than charting only after the care is given. Problem-oriented charting may use other formats but still be considered a problem-solving approach.

Date/ Time	Problem Number	
0800		S—I feel fine this morning. I don't hurt anywhere right now. O—Awake, alert, oriented X3. PERLA. Eupneic. Lung sounds clear. Pulse strong, regular all extremities. Skin pink, warm, dry. Abd. dressing dry & intact. No other skin lesions noted. Ambulated to bath by self. J. Duffy, RN
0930	4	S—I have a dull pain where I had that surgery. I would rather try some medicine by mouth instead of a shot. O—Frowning. Holding abdomen. A—Alteration in comfort: pain in incisional area related to surgical trauma. P—Oral analgesic per order. I—Tylenol #3 P.O. ————————————— J. Duffy, RN
1015		E—States pain relieved ————————————— J. Duffy, RN

Figure 11.2: SOAPIE nurses' notes.

Variations of Problem-Oriented Charting

Variations of the SOAP format are used in problem-oriented charting. There may be some differences in the overall approach of the data base and problem list. The same type of general planning may be used, but the progress notes may use a different format. Two variations of progress notes, APIE and ADIE, are discussed in the following paragraphs.

APIE

A slight variation of the problem-oriented nurses record is called APIE. This is very similar to the SOAPIE format but combines some of the items. The subjective and objective data are combined with the nursing diagnosis in the first part, "A." The remainder of this format, PIE, follows the SOAPIE format in listing a plan, the implementation, and the evaluation. The 0800 assessment is similar to the narrative format, with the subjective and objective data together. Since the assessment is essentially normal, a nursing diagnosis is not necessary. The 0930 and 1015 entries are shown in Figure 11.3.

0930	A—Frowning, holding abdomen. c/o dull pain in incisional area. Requested oral pain medication. Alteration in comfort: pain in incisional area related to surgical trama. P—Oral analgesic per order. I—Demerol 50mg ⁱᵉʳʳᵒʳ JD I—Tylenol #3 P.O. ————————————— J. Duffy RN
1015	E—States pain relieved ————————————— J. Duffy, RN

Figure 11.3: APIE nurses' notes.

ADIE

Another proposed approach is termed ADIE (pronounced addy to rhyme with caddy.) It suggests that a modified nursing care plan be used as a part of the permanent record. The nursing care plan lists the nursing diagnoses with plans for meeting the unmet needs as specified by the diagnoses. Potential problems are included to alert the health care personnel to monitor specific aspects of the patient's condition. Dates on which each nursing diagnosis was identified and resolved as well as a goal, or outcome criteria, which includes a time frame, are incorporated in the plan. Resolved diagnoses are highlighted to remain a legible part of the record for reference in the event of a recurrence.

This method separates medical and nursing approaches and does not make nursing diagnoses secondary to medical diagnoses. With the care plan a part of the patient chart, directing documentation toward the plan is more readily accomplished and the nursing diagnoses can be referred to by number or an abbreviated form. The charting format includes the following items.

A—Assessment
D—Diagnosis (Nursing Diagnosis)
I—Implementation
E—Evaluation

The **assessment** includes the objective and the subjective data. While it is vital that the nurse be able to differentiate the two, they are facets of a total patient assessment. Separating the two types of data in documentation increases the possibility of repetition, which is time-consuming and confusing. Subjective data is indicated as such by the use of quotation marks or preceded by "states . ." to provide clarity.

Documentation using a narrative style with subjective and objective data together in the assessment facilitates analysis of the data to prepare for the next step in ADIE. This approach suggests the use of a flow sheet to decrease the amount of time and effort spent in documentation. Any abnormal assessment noted on the flow sheet requires the attention of the nurse and should be further documented.

The **nursing diagnosis** is based on the data in the assessment. It may be noted in an abbreviated form on the nurses' notes as it is recorded on the care plan. For example, "Alteration in comfort: pain in incisional area related to surgical trauma" would appear on the nursing care plan but might be written as "Pain in incisional area" with or without a number referring to the care plan when documented in the nurses' progress notes.

Implementation is the next logical step in the process. This step is recorded in telegraphic style, just as in the assessment. The plan is omitted because it is part of the nursing care plan on the chart and would be redundant. The time constraints placed on the nurse are real and must be considered in determining the amount of documentation necessary to reflect continuity of care.

Recording nursing actions after they have been completed is based on a recognized principle of charting—documentation after the fact. Documentation of patient care is what the nurse has done with/to/for the patient, not what the nurse plans to do. This also follows current payment practices of insurance companies.

They often utilize nurses' notes to determine the payment to be made based on care the patient actually received and not what was planned. Legally, courts are interested in what was done, not what was planned. Plans without written notation of implementation are invitations for lawsuits based on errors of omission. The implementation in the ADIE format documents what has been done to resolve the nursing diagnosis by following the care plan previously developed.

The **evaluation** of the care implemented is the final portion of the ADIE format. Was the action taken effective in resolving the nursing diagnosis? If so, should it be continued? If not, can the reason be pinpointed? What modifications are suggested to attain the goals specified in the care plan? The evaluation might be simple statement to note that a medication given for pain was effective or might be in more detail.

Figure 11.4 is an example of charting the same situation as before but following the ADIE format and using the 0930 and 1015 entries only, as in the APIE example.

0930	A—Frowning, holding abd. States dull pain in incisional area. Requested oral pain medication
	D—#5. Pain incisional area
	I—Tylenol #3 P.O. ————————— J. Duffy, RN
1015	E—States pain relieved. Resting quietly. ————————— J. Duffy, RN

Figure 11.4: ADIE nurses' notes.

In each of these charting examples, the same data is recorded. All are acceptable methods. In general, problem-oriented charting is a patient-centered, problem-solving approach that follows the premises of the nursing process. If the POMR format as originally established is utilized, nursing concerns are secondary to medical. Many health care facilities use a SOAPIE type format with the nursing progress record separated from the medical. The ADIE format further separates the medical and nursing approaches. In the application of any of the problem-solving formats, some health care agencies may prefer to have labeled columns for each of the components included. The charting will be the same, the only difference being the placement on the page. Regardless of the manner of recording data, nurses must use the format of the facility in which they practice.

FLOW SHEETS

Most health care agencies use flow sheets of one type or another. Graphic sheets for recording vital signs are the oldest form of flow sheets. Other information such as intake and output has gradually been included on these. In the past 10 to 15 years, the information recorded on flow sheets has increased tremendously in an effort to reduce the time required to document nursing care.

The information recorded on, and general format of, flow sheets vary. Some are a checklist type but need additional nurses' notes. Others have space to make a limited number of individual notations as part of the checklist. A few tend to serve more as a reminder of items to chart, with space for brief notes on the form. In some health care agencies, only routine procedures such as hygienic measures and meals are recorded on flow sheets. Many flow sheets have a column for each shift. Just as with the format used to record nurses' notes, no one flow sheet is right and others wrong.

Advantages and Disadvantages

Some nurses are beginning to criticize the widespread use of flow sheets, especially the checklist type. The argument is that their use tends to reduce the amount of communication with patients, since the nurse enters the room with a checklist in hand and limits questions to those on the list.

However, the use of checklists may not be the problem, but the *way* in which they are used. Care must be taken not to depend on flow sheets for all charting. Problems need to be recorded in detail, but the data on flow sheets does not need to be repeated in the nurses' notes. This defeats the purpose of the flow sheet. The timesaving factor of flow sheets makes them a definite positive factor in agencies in which there is a shortage of personnel. Like many things, the proper application is the key to effectiveness.

Special Flow Sheets

Several special types of checklists are available for different purposes. These can be quite useful. Forms for recording vital signs that must be taken frequently, critical intake and output records, and preoperative checklists are a few examples. Emergency rooms have developed special checklists that not only reduce the amount of time necessary in documenting assessments but also serve as a reminder of assessments to be made in trauma situations. Outpatient surgery units and obstetrical units may have special checklists pertinent to the focus of the service.

Daily Care Flow Sheets

Figures 11.5 through 11.7 are examples of portions of three types of flow sheets. These show only items included in "Activity" and "Safety." There are other categories included in the assessments, as well as spaces in which to record routine care. A comparison will illustrate the variations in the amount of information that is entered with initials or a check mark. Initialing each space is preferable, since it is impossible to determine who made a check mark.

Each type of flow sheet in Figures 11.5 through 11.7 will have advantages and disadvantages. No one form is considered the ultimate answer by all health care agencies. These examples show only one column. Most will have a column for each shift.

Activity	Level of immobility	Comp[ ] Partial[√] Up ad lib[ ]
	Type of activity	Bd[ ] Ch[√] Amb[ ] Dgl[ ]
	How accomplished	Self[ ] Asst[√]
	Range of motion	Active[ ] Passive[ ] Full[ ]
Safety	Side rails up	Yes[√] No[ ]
	Call light in reach	Yes[√] No[ ]
	Bed position	Hi[ ] Low[√]
	Restraints on	NA[√] Body[ ] Vest[ ] Wrist[ ]

Figure 11.5: Checklist-type flow sheet.

Activity	Range of motion	Full[R] Partial[L] Passive L 10⁰⁰ JD
	Type activity	Chr[√] Amb[ ] Self[ ] Asst[ ]
	Toleration	Time 1030 Response 1 hr. JD
	Reposition	Self[ ] q 2 hrs JD
Safety	Side rails up	x 4 Check q 2 hrs JD
	Call light in reach	No[ ] Yes[√] Check q 2 h JD
	Bed position	Hi[ ] Lo[√] JD
	Restraints	Type NA Check

Figure 11.6: Flow sheet with limited space for notations.

Activity	Range of motion	Active R–Passive L–10⁰⁰ JD
	Type activity	Chair–assist – 1030 x 1 hr JD
	Toleration	Slips down if not propped up JD
	Repositioned	q 2 h JD
Safety	Side rails up	x 4 ck. q 2 h JD
	Call light in reach	R side–ck q 2 h JD
	Bed position	Low except during care JD
	Restraints	N.A.

Figure 11.7: Flow sheet that serves as reminder.

These are brief excerpts from different types of flow sheets. There is always a place for the date and the signature of the nurse, even when entries are initialed. There may be a space for the initials used by the nurse, along with the nurses' full signature at the bottom of the flow sheet. Many flow sheets include a space at the bottom or on the reverse side for progress notes so that all of the day's data can be on a single sheet. On flow sheets in which there is ample space for writing, the nurse usually notes the time with initials indicating when procedures were performed or status checked. There are myriad variations on each type of flow sheet.

CHARTING SHORT BUT SMART

Time is always of the essence in bedside nursing. Since the time required for charting is a frequent complaint of nurses, the solution seems to be in the direction of reducing the amount of time necessary to adequately document all pertinent data on each patient.

Flow Sheets The flow sheets discussed are timesavers but should not be relied on too heavily. Those with space in which to write individual notes can be used very effectively. This is where the nurse can chart smart. Anything already noted on the flow sheet should not be repeated. Any abnormal assessments noted on the assessment will need further clarification, but if assessments covered in the flow sheets are normal, there is no need to repeat.

Working Notes Keeping a pocket notebook for working notes has been mentioned. This reduces "thinking" time but is a bit of repetition, since the nurse is writing items twice, even though the working notes are very brief. Some health care agencies have printouts of the patient census, with spaces for noting special procedures. This enables the nurse to make notes readily. Some facilities allow the nurse to place the current day's note pages on a clipboard for easy access.

Care Plans A good nursing care plan can be a basis for easier charting. Documentation of patient care should relate to the care plan. By referring to the plan, the nurse is made aware of items that need to be charted. Documentation should follow through, with evaluation directed toward nursing actions suggested by the care plan.

Developing Own Approach Using telegraphic style in all charting is a timesaver in the reduction of words. Saying exactly what is meant in the fewest possible words is the goal. Each nurse develops a particular style of charting and uses those suggestions that are of the grestest benefit. The nurse should know the hospital policy and adhere to its rules. Chart as often as is specified and in the manner recommended. Charting may seem a necessary evil, but it becomes easier with time. It is truly a safeguard for the conscientious nurse.

USE OF COMPUTERS IN HEALTH CARE FACILITIES

The use of computers in documenting patient care is in its infancy, but, like all infants, it will grow. Computers are being used rather widely in health care agencies for census lists, for sending requisitions to various departments, and for recording laboratory results. They are used extensively in the business offices. Their application in pharmacy departments is proving invaluable. Many programs show safe dosage parameters for individual medications, cross-reference drug interactions, and alert the pharmacist if a drug allergy is noted on the patient data. There are a number of computer programs on diagnosis and treatment of various medical conditions that physicians are finding valuable.

Documenting Patient Care on Computers

The inception of computer usage in documenting patient care has progressed rather slowly. Programs are becoming available that should be the most valuable timesaver yet available to nurses in the realm of record keeping. Some of the

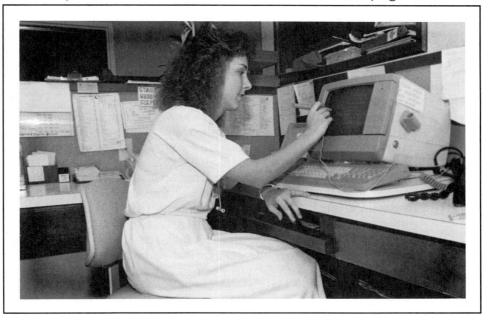

programs are set up with parameters for assessment, which the nurse checks in a fashion similar to detailed flow sheets. These have the advantage of preventing an oversight by the nurse. However, much like the criticism of the detailed flow sheets, this could take away some of the individualization. Some programs leave more room for the nurses' input.

An enormous plus is the advent of care plans on computer softwear. From the assessment data, the computer derives a care plan that can be printed out readily. These are standardized care plans written for one specific nursing diagnosis or for multiple diagnoses, such as a postoperative care plan. They are readily adapted to the individual patient. Some of these care plans are goal oriented and give outcome criteria with suggestions for nursing interventions. Some have options from which to choose, some allow for individual data input, and some are a combination. Programs may allow for evaluation, with automatic modification of the plan when indicated.

Computerized documentation has proved to be a great asset when used in auditing quality of care in an agency. As computer applications in nursing increase, there will be a greater need for standardization of the terminology used and the data collected in assessments.

Questions on Usage

Computer programs continue to become more sophisticated, but there are some questions that are frequently posed regarding their usage in documenting patient care. One area concerns the confidentiality of the records and the patient's right to privacy. Programs are available that necessitate an access code to obtain patient information, but many people still question the possibility of hackers breaking the code. Even with safeguards, the nurse has the responsibility of protecting the confidentially of the patient. Refraining from documenting non-health related information and refusing to let an unauthorized person know anything about accessing the records is a step toward safeguarding.

Another concern that has been expressed is the possibility of accidentally erasing records. A safeguard is built into programs to prevent accidental erasure as well as to prevent anything from being changed in the record once it has been entered. As computer technology advances, more reliable safeguards will be developed.

Possible Future of Computers in Health Care Facilities

The use of computers in our society is a fact of life that will become more and more a part of everyday activities. Just as many people resisted the introduction of machinery to speed up production, so many people will continue to resist the use of computers. It is true that in some areas machines tended to make the old idea of craftsmanship obsolete, but with proper application these machines retained the value of the craftsman and added new dimensions to the art. So with computers.

Many health care personnel now oppose the use of computers in documenting patient care with the argument that they tend to depersonalize the patient. It is not the computer but the user that commits the error. Computers are definitely timesavers but require common sense in the proper application in patient care. They cannot take the place of the compassionate nurse at the bedside or make professional decisions regarding care of the patient.

Computers may not come into widespread use in hospitals until it becomes economically feasible to have a minicomputer for each patient. For computers to be used to record all aspects of patient care, it would necessitate computerized physician orders. The picture of physicians waiting their turn to write orders does not fit the current picture in the health care scene. With individual computers, the application would be comparable to the current use of the patient chart.

The possibility of computers in patient rooms is being explored, but many questions will have to be answered and standards established for the general use of computers in maintaining patient records. How would errors in charting be corrected? How would late entries be made? How would patient care be affected if the computers were down? How well can the data be protected from unauthorized persons? Could there be sufficient safeguards to prevent changes in data entered? The future will have to answer these and many as yet unasked questions. There is little doubt, however, that the role of computers will continue to grow in our society, including the area of documentation of patient care.

As noted previously, no one way of charting is right and the others wrong. The perfect method has not been developed. Institutions have their preferred methods, but even these are not static. Progressive health care agencies may make changes relatively often, as new concepts are tried. Flow sheets are being used in varying degrees, and computer charting is being instituted in some places. Nursing may eventually arrive at a uniform approach. However, regardless of the future approaches to documenting nursing care, the basic principles will remain relatively the same. The fact remains that good charting is good communication.

IN A CAPSULE

The use of *correct medical terminology* enables professionals to communicate more effectively. The use of *clinical terms with patients* should be limited to those that the nurse is certain are familiar to the patient. Medical *abbreviations* can be misinterpreted unless personnel adhere to the agency's list of those acceptable.

Information recorded in nurses' notes includes *subjective and objective observations* and all *actions of the nurse.* The *principles of charting* should be observed in all documentation of patient care.

Nurses' notes must be *accurate* in all details.

It is essential that the notes are *complete*, with all pertinent data included.

Only *factual* information should be recorded, with no conclusions or labels.

Language should be *clear,* with the use of specific medical terms.

Writing *concise* notes using telegraphic style saves time for the writer and the reader.

Charting must be kept *current*.

Nurses' notations must be *technically correct* to be acceptable legally.

The order style of nurses' notes is termed *narrative* because it does not follow a particular order. *Problem-oriented* records are a patient-centered, problem-solving approach that indicates the nursing care plan and is consistent with the premises of the nursing process. Problem-oriented nurses' notes may use a *SOAPIE, APIE,* or *ADIE* format. *Flow sheets* are effective timesavers but must be used in conjunction with more detailed notes.

The nurse can *chart "smart and short"* by effectively using flow sheets, making working notes, utilizing well-written care plans, and using telegraphic style with no repetition of information. *Computer charting* may be the future method of documenting patient care, but the principles and approaches will remain relatively the same.

DO YOU REMEMBER

- the primary reason for using correct medical terminology?
- the advantage and the danger in the use of abbreviations?
- the categories of information that nurses chart?
- at least five of the seven principles of charting discussed?
- the general approach of problem-oriented medical records?
- the four parts of problem-oriented medical records?
- what is included in each part of the SOAPIER format?

- the profits and pitfalls of flow sheets?
- timesaving approaches to effective charting?

CAN YOU DESCRIBE

- the terminology you would use to explain a complicated procedure to a patient?
- a technically correct nurses' entry on a patient chart?
- a well-written narrative nurses' note?
- the rationale given for the use of the ADIE format in preference to the SOAPIE or APIE format?

ACTION, PLEASE

1. Use the following patient situation to complete the excerpt of the following flow sheet. Only those items relevant to the situation are included. Assume that a graphic sheet is included, on which vital signs are charted, that there is a column before the one shown on the flow sheet with space for the night nurse to chart, and that a space is at the bottom for your signature. Record the nurses' progress notes in at least two of the formats discussed.

Mr. Barber was hospitalized with pneumonia 2 days ago. This morning he is coughing up large amounts of thick, yellow mucus. Oxygen is continuous at 3L/m. His respiration was 24 and shallow before respiratory therapy by the technician. Following the treatment, his respiration was 18 and deeper. He appeared weak and needed assistance with his bath. He stated that he felt much better after the bath and therapy.

Flow sheet:

Date		0700–1500
	Lung sounds	
Respiratory	Cough/Results	
	Therapy/Results	
	Oxygen therapy	

Safety	Side rails Up _____	_____
	Call light in reach	_____
	Bed position _____	_____
	Restraints _____	_____
	Other _____	_____
Hygiene	Bath _____	_____
	Back care _____	_____
	Oral care _____	_____
	Other _____	_____

Time	Nurses' Progress Notes
_____	_____
_____	_____
_____	_____
_____	_____
_____	_____
_____	_____
_____	_____
_____	_____
_____	_____
_____	_____
_____	_____
_____	_____
_____	_____
_____	_____
_____	_____
_____	_____

2. *How Would You Document It?* While you were bathing Mrs. Toler, you noticed a redened area about the size of a silver dollar over the sacral area. You massaged the area, positioned her on the right side, and reminded her to stay off her back.

Consider the following nurses' progress notes. Determine which principle or principles each notation violates.

a. Decubitus over sacral area. Massaged. Turned.

    _____

    _____

b. Noticed a small reddened area on patient's sacral area during bath. Turned. Told to stay on side.

    _____

    _____

c. 4 cm reddened area over sacrum. Massaged. Positioned R side. Instructed to turn side to side q2h.

    _____

    _____

d. Pt. has 4 cm red area over sacrum. Told her not to lie on back. Massaged sacral area. Left on R side.

    _____

    _____

Chart the same information using narrative and SOAP formats.

_____

_____

_____

_____

_____

_____

UNIT III BIBLIOGRAPHY

Afflerbach, Denise. A Flow Sheet that Saves Time and Trouble. *RN*, January, 1986.

Apse, Aina and Stetler, Cheryl B. Avoiding Terms of Bewilderment. *Nursing 85*. December.

Bergerson, Stephen R. More About Charting with a Jury in Mind. *Nursing 88*, April.

Bernzweig, Eli P. Go on Record with Nothing But the Truth. *RN*, April, 1985.

Boatwright, Debbie and Crumette, Beauty D. How to Plan and Conduct a Patient Care Conference. *Nursing 87*, December.

Bradley, Jean C. and Edinberg, Mark A. *Communication in the Nursing Context*, Second Edition. Norwalk, Connecticut: Appleton-Century-Crofts, 1986.

Brooke, Penny S. Will the Law Let You Keep a Patient's Secrets? *RN*, August 1987.

Carlson, Robert E. *The Nurse's Guide to Better Communication*. Glenview, Illinois: Scott, Foresman and Company, 1984.

Cohen, Michael R. Play It Safe. *Nursing 82*, October. (Reprint *Nursing 87*, July.)

Cook, Margo. *Computerized Quality Assurance: Documentation, Nursing Diagnosis and Audit.* Paper presented at the 2nd National Conference on Computer Technology and Nursing held at the National Institutes of Health on July 2, 1982.

Cormier, L. Sherilyn, et al. *Interviewing and Helping Skills for Health Professionals.* Monterey, California: Wadsworth Health Sciences Division, 1984.

Ellis, Janice R. and Nowlis, Elizabeth A. *Nursing: A Human Needs Approach*, Third Edition. Boston: Houghton Mifflin Company, 1985.

Fritz, Paul A., et al. *Interpersonal Communication in Nursing.* Norwalk, Connecticut: Appleton-Century-Crofts, 1984.

Kelly, Lucie Young. *Dimensions of Professional Nursing*, Fifth Edition. New York: Macmillan Publishing Company, 1985.

Kerr, Avice H. How the Write Stuff Can Go Wrong. *Nursing 87*, January.

Kozier, Barbara and Erb, Glenora. *Fundamentals of Nursing: Concepts and Procedures.* Third Edition. Menlo Park, California: Addison-Wesley Publishing Company, 1987.

Light, Nancy L. *Developing a Hospital Information System Nursing Data Base: A Pragmatic Approach.* Paper presented at the 2nd National Conference on Computer Technology and Nursing held at the National Institutes of Health on July 2, 1982.

Miller, Mary J. *ADIE: A "Mightier Pen" for Documentation.* Manuscript submitted for publication, 1988.

Narrow, Barbara W. and Buschle, Kay B. *Fundamentals of Nursing Practice.* New York: John Wiley and Sons, 1987.

Northop, Cynthia E. Filling In Charting Gaps . . . In Court. *Nursing 87*, September.

Northouse, Peter G. and Northouse, Laurel L. *Health Communication.* Englewood Cliffs, New Jersey: Prentice-Hall, Inc., 1985.

Philpott, Mary. 20 Rules for Good Charting. *Nursing 86*, August.

Rich, Paula L. Make the Most of Your Charting Time. *Nursing 83*, March. (Reprint *Nursing 87*, May.)

Rich, Paula L. With This Flow Sheet, Less Is More. *Nursing 85*, July.

Saperstein, Arlyn B. and Frazier, Margaret A. *Introduction to Nursing Practice.* Philadelphia: F. A. Davis Company, 1980.

Sathre, Freda S., et al. *Let's Talk*, Second Edition. Glenview, Illinois: Scott, Foresman and Company, 1977.

Scher, Betty B. Are Checklists Replacing Good Care? *Nursing 88*, January.

Shaughnessy, Allen F. It's Medspeak to us, but Greek to them. *RN*, December, 1987.

Smith, Carole E. Upgrade Your Shift Reports with the Three R's. *Nursing 86*. February.

Weaver, Richard L., II. *Understanding Interpersonal Communication*, Fourth Edition. Glenview, Illinois: Scott, Foresman and Company, 1987.

INDEX